I Choose to Live!

Beverly D. Brown

Sat. Nov 3, 1990 at Dillons Book Store.

To Edna, With love. All my best wishes. God Bless! Beverly Brown

WD

TO SOW THE FALLOW SOIL

Winston-Derek Publishers, Inc.
Pennywell Drive—P.O. Box 90883
Nashville, TN 37209

First printing

The names of some persons and places have been changed to protect their identities. This work details the experiences of those involved, but is not intended to be used as a guide to self-treatment. Readers should consult their physicians before using any described treatment, exercise or diet. Anyone suspecting lupus should contact a doctor, preferably a rheumatologist.

PUBLISHED BY WINSTON-DEREK PUBLISHERS, INC.
Nashville, Tennessee 37205

Library of Congress Catalog Card No: 89-50710
ISBN: 1-55523-232-9

Printed in the United States of America

With love to my children,
Adrienne, Jeff and Annie

Contents

Foreword

This intense book portrays the author's physical and emotional impression of her chronic illness. Although she has written specifically about systemic lupus erythematosus (SLE), many patients with any type of chronic illness can identify with the suffering and the dilemmas they must face before the diagnosis is made, as well as throughout the entire treatment.

The author has covered the broad spectrum of the treatment and approach to chronic illness—lifestyle, diet, rehabilitation modalities—each of which may help provide relief from their suffering. This book is also a source of extremely pertinent information for all health professionals to aid in understanding the plight of a patient with a chronic illness such as SLE.

In addition, I should mention that persons who have never experienced chronic illness will appreciate and benefit from the author's story. Written with a great deal of warmth and feeling, it will involve the reader from the beginning of a struggle with a devastating chronic disease to the triumphant acceptance.

I take great pleasure in highly recommending this book.

GIDEON DARVISH, M.D.
Co-director, Arthritis Rehabilitation Program
Daniel Freeman Memorial Hospital
Inglewood, California

Preface

About one in 500 Americans has lupus. It is more common than leukemia, muscular dystrophy or multiple sclerosis. The symptoms can occur in any part of the body and vary from mild to life-threatening.

I Choose to Live is the true story of my terrifying experience with the chronic illness, lupus. I sincerely hope that it will help others who still suffer from loneliness, despair and misdiagnosis. There is a solution.

Acknowledgments

A large number of people provided their expertise and knowledge and touched my life during the time that I was writing this book. To all of them I offer my deep appreciation and sincere gratitude.

I am particularly grateful to my dear friend, Parks Herzog, for his constant help and encouragement.

I would also like to express my special thanks to the members of the lupus rap groups who so willingly shared their experiences.

God grant me the
Serenity
to accept the things
I cannot change,
the Courage
to change the things I can,
and the Wisdom
to know the difference.

Reinhold Niebuhr

1
Illness in Paradise

It was a warm October morning in 1974 and from my tenth-floor office window I could see the reflection of the sun on the ocean. Even though I had been living in Honolulu for almost a year, its beauty continued to fascinate me. I can't believe I'm actually here, I thought with a smile. My life is good. It's exciting. This is indeed my paradise.

I glanced at my watch. Nearly ten o'clock. It was almost time to deliver the morning report. I sighed and reluctantly turned my chair back toward the desk and adjusted my new Island hairdo, perky and short for swimming. As I checked the time again, my vision blurred momentarily when I tried to focus on the numbers. Too much weekend sun yesterday, I reasoned, or maybe it was the paint fumes. They had been redecorating my office for several days. Oh, well, sun or paint, it would pass. Back to work.

At five-foot six I weighed only 120 pounds, but it was amazingly hard to lift my aching body. As I approached the first secretary's desk, a sudden wave of dizziness made me grab the nearest chair to keep from falling. Everything was spinning around me. I sat down quickly. I'd been feeling weak and queasy all morning, but now a strange feeling of numbness came over me. I had difficulty breathing.

"Are you all right?" my boss, Robert Morgan, asked.

"I don't know," I stammered. Several secretaries

had come over to see what was wrong. "I think I can stand up now." I was too embarrassed to admit how wobbly my legs were and hoped that I could walk. As others approached I felt more and more uncomfortable. Why didn't they all go away?

"Go see the doctor across the street," Mr. Morgan advised. "I'll send someone with you."

"No," I responded after thinking a moment. "But thanks anyway. If it's all right, I'll just grab a cab and go home. I think it's the paint fumes. I'm sure I'll be okay by tomorrow." Actually, I wasn't sure about anything except that I wanted to get home and lie down.

The cab arrived to take me to my apartment at the Ilikai Hotel. On the way, I thought about my plans for the evening. I'd be seeing Glen, and as usual that was something I looked forward to. Dear Glen, tall and with that rustic look I found so appealing, had taken charge of my life. An expert in electronics, a retired naval officer and now owner of an electronics company in Honolulu, Glen was a man used to being in command of people. We had met a short time after my move to the Island, and in just six breathtaking months he had become important and special to me, an indispensable part of my life.

"Bev, I love you," he had said a lifetime ago, and again last night. Remembering his words sent a warm feeling through my body. Hawaii still appeared as a miracle to me. So did Glen. "Am I in love?" was my constant question.

The taxi pulled up in front of the Ilikai. As I walked through the expansive, elegant lobby I saw a bellboy holding the elevator open for me. He smiled and followed me in.

"What's wrong?" he asked when he saw me lean against the wall.

"I think I had too much sun yesterday," I said, trying to dispel the panic in his eyes.

"Don't faint! Maybe you'd better see the doctor. He's right on the mezzanine. Okay? I'll push the button for you."

"I guess so," I said hesitantly. It probably wasn't anything to worry about, but I did feel awful. Perhaps the doctor could help.

Although I always wore a hat in the sun, lately it had seemed as though being in the sun made me feel sick afterwards. So I'd been protecting myself more than usual. Could it really just be too much sun? Years later I would learn how close to the truth this was.

I'd been to the beach yesterday with Marilyn, my special and beautiful Hawaii friend. It had started out a perfect day—warm sun, calm water, just enough waves to make it fun to swim in. But when we jumped up from the sand laughing, and raced to the water, my body felt strangely heavy and weak. As I entered the water, it got even worse, and suddenly I could hardly move and had to lie on my back to keep afloat. I'd made it back to shore, collapsing on the sand, then home, to bed. "Just a little tired today," I'd lied to Marilyn. "And I feel a little dizzy, that's all."

The elevator opened at the mezzanine, and I went into the empty waiting room. "It'll be just a few minutes," the receptionist informed me. "Please have a seat."

I walked over to the chair, sat down and passed out.

Consciousness returned slowly. I was lying on an examining table, my vision blurry and a ringing in my ears. I turned my head to see the nurse standing by my side. Next to her was a man wearing a white medical jacket.

"Mrs. Brown," he said. "I'm Dr. Burns. You are in my office. How are you feeling now?"

"Tired," I answered, squinting at him. "What happened?"

"You lost consciousness," he said. "Out in the waiting room, then again on the table here. Don't you remember!"

"Yes," I said, smiling up at him. "I remember. It's all very strange, but I feel a little better now."

"Can you sit up?"

I nodded my head. "I'll be all right." I sat there feeling weak and dizzy.

After a brief examination, the diagnosis was "viral infection."

"I'm going to give you some antibiotics," Dr. Burns said. "Don't do too much the next few days and you should be fine by the weekend. But continue taking the pills for ten days."

Don't do too much! He had to be kidding; I could barely stand up. I moved very slowly on the way to my apartment on the sixth floor. The phone was ringing when I got there.

"Darn," I said, kicking the locked door with my foot while fumbling for my keys. "Open, open," I said. My purse dropped to the floor and the contents scattered. Tears rolled down my face. Oh—there it was, the lost key. It went easily into the lock, and I made my way inside, quickly lifting the phone.

"Hello." I gasped, falling into a chair.

"Bev?" Glen questioned. "is that you? Are you okay?"

"Yes," I said weakly. "Just out of breath."

"What's wrong?" he asked. I could hear the concern in his voice. "I called your office and they said you went home ill."

I looked at the mess out in the hall. "It's nothing serious," I sniffed. "Just the flu. The doctor says I'll be fine in a few days."

"Then why are you crying?"

"I dropped my purse on the floor trying to get in to

answer the phone."

"Oh. I was worried."

"I'm sorry. Hang on a minute. I need a cigarette." I gathered up my purse and its scattered contents and returned to the phone. "I'm back now. Sorry I worried you. I'm feeling better already."

"What a relief. The girl at your switchboard sounded so vague, like you had an accident or something."

This was no fun. I wanted a little sympathy. Didn't he know how sick I felt?

"Well," I began, with just enough hesitation to evoke guilt in Genghis Khan, "I did sort of pass out." I heard Glen gasp; that was more like it. "But I'm better now, really," I said. I wanted him to know how brave I was being. "The doctor says I will be all right by the weekend."

"How about dinner?" Glen suggested. "Are you well enough to eat out or shall I bring over some Chinese food?"

The thought of food..."Thanks, but I don't think so," I said. "I'm going to crawl into bed. Maybe that's the best thing to do." I made a few lighthearted remarks to convince him that I would be all right and promised to phone in the morning.

I returned to work the following week, but I still couldn't function. "How about a few more days rest?" Mr. Morgan suggested.

"Thanks, but I'll be fine," I said. At eleven o'clock I went home. Everything was whirling around me. My ears were still ringing, as if they were pressed between two seashells.

The spinning in my head and the off-balance sensation persisted. I couldn't leave my apartment for fear of falling. Most of the time I was too weak to even get out of bed. For the next seven days I felt as if I were going up and down in an elevator. I was feverish, and there was a constant ache throughout my body that made it difficult to sleep, even though I was desperately tired. Glen had been over every day and wanted me to go back to the doctor. I refused. I could handle this myself.

One morning I woke up barely able to move. I was aching all over and my entire body felt swollen. It was as if there were a huge mass growing inside me and pushing to get out. My neck was stiff and my arms and legs felt heavy. The pain was excruciating. I phoned Glen. When he arrived, he insisted on calling the doctor then and there. I listened as he explained my symptoms over the phone.

"The nurse said to come down." Glen relayed, hanging up the phone and walking towards me in one movement. "The doctor will see you right now."

He gave me my robe and took my hand to help me out of bed. "Okay, okay," I said, louder than I had planned. I was beginning to become irritated by the whole business. I hated being sick, and most of all I was embarrassed to have Glen see me like this.

"Sorry, I didn't mean to yell," I said. "I'm just so tired of all this. I can't understand why I'm still so sick. The doctor said a few days. It's been weeks and I feel worse!"

"I know, honey," he responded, holding me close for a brief moment. "It's been going on too long. Let's find out what the problem is."

With Glen's help I made it downstairs to the doctor's office. I was immediately taken to an examining room while Glen disappeared back into the waiting room. The nurse handed me one of those gowns that opens either in the front or the back, depending on which side of the body is to be pushed and prodded. These must have been designed by a sadistic male chauvinist, bent on humiliating and embarrassing the entire female population, I thought. Or did men have to wear these too? I was too weak to get out of my robe and couldn't focus my eyes on anything. I put up my hands to steady my spinning head. I was so dizzy that I couldn't even identify the wall painting a few feet away. What was it, anyway? I squinted to try to bring the picture into focus, but to no avail. I felt more comfortable sitting up than lying down, and then found that I couldn't sit there very long without falling over. So when the nurse went out, I lay on my side and curled my legs up under me, waiting for the doctor. I choked back the tears that had started to fill my eyes. Doctor, please hurry, I silently prayed. I heard the door open.

After a brief examination Dr. Burns said, with that rare warmth that doctors usually save for the family of the deceased, "You look extremely tired."

I could imagine what I looked like. Why did he think I was here, anyway? Actually I was grateful that he took me seriously and agreed with the way I was feeling.

"I'd like you to see an ear, nose and throat specialist. In fact, I think we should admit you to the hospital and find out what's going on."

I was relieved that someone was thinking. I certainly couldn't. It was all I could do to lift my head off the pillow.

He called an ambulance and I was taken to Straub hospital. I had convinced Glen to go back to work, with my promise to phone him as soon as I was settled in a room. I was too ill to be scared, but something was bothering me. Something I couldn't quite remember. Hadn't I been through a similar situation before, or was my mind playing tricks on me? Was it *deja vu*? Then it came back to me.

It was in 1965, nine years before, during my second marriage. For several weeks I'd had a persistent cold and a low-grade fever. I'd lost thirty pounds in one month. My neck was stiff then, too, and my body ached all over. The doctor had diagnosed the Asian flu and I was given antibiotics and instructions to go to bed for a few days, just like this time. But the cold and fever persisted. Then one day I woke up in severe pain, so weak I could hardly move. I reached over to call the doctor, and the room spun around as I knocked over the phone. My husband came in and dialed the doctor, then handed me the phone.

"Mrs. Brown, I think you should come in to the office," Dr. Morris said. I couldn't move and told him so. I'll never forget his words and the sarcasm in his voice. "You mean if there was a fire you couldn't get out of bed?"

It sounded so silly, but I didn't think I could. "All right," I'd said, "I'll come by this afternoon." Instead, I'd ended up in the hospital that time too. Then the symptoms went away, and I never did know what had happened. No diagnosis. I'd chalked it up as a bad case of the flu.

Now I really began to worry, and I didn't know these doctors, this hospital so far from home. Maybe I should call my family. No, no—wait till you find out what is wrong. Maybe it's nothing. Don't call them yet.

At the hospital they got me settled in my room, and later Glen came to visit, bringing his love and comfort. How good it was to have him there! Soon I'd be seeing the specialist; soon I'd find out something.

The next morning I explained my symptoms to the ear, nose and throat doctor, a Dr. Woodbury. He nodded his head and read aloud from my chart. " 'Progressive lethargy and dizziness. Experiencing a sense of fullness in her head and a sensation of pressure in her ears.' That sounds like what you've told me."

"Yes, and sometimes if I force the air out through my nose while I hold it tightly, the pressure will be relieved," I explained. "This dizzy feeling comes and goes, day and night. I can't control it—there's nothing I can do. Also, I'm very tired and my vision is blurry all the time. It's really hard to focus." I took a deep breath, letting all the air out in one comforting sigh. That was a load off my mind. Maybe I should allow a tear or two. No, mustn't do that.

"It seems as though there is a disturbance of the balancing mechanism, the labyrinth, in your inner ear," the doctor said. "Many things could cause this, and I want to run some tests. The symptoms are similar to those of Meniere's disease, and I want to rule that out." He saw my questioning look and went on to explain that Meniere's is a disease of the inner ear that can follow an infection such as I had.

"Disabling dizziness and ringing in the ears is quite common," he continued. "However, left untreated, it could result in partial deafness. We'll check that out tomorrow or the next day. But first you need some rest."

True to his word, he allowed me several days to rest, with the help of pain killers and sleeping pills. Then the probing began. As each test proved normal, I was whisked off for another. Between the flurry of tests, x-rays, examinations, having blood drawn, and a constant flow of medicines, I became numbed to what was happening. I just went along with it all, praying that a solution could be found.

They couldn't find anything wrong, but I knew I was sick, really sick. What did the doctors think? Why couldn't they find something? Anything! Just give this incubus a name!

After a few more days of rest, I left the hospital, with all the tests still inconclusive. Further tests could be done as an out-patient. I'd had enough of hospitals. I just wanted to go home.

Several days later Dr. Woodbury sent me to an outside lab for a very sophisticated test, an electronystagmogram.

"You might experience some discomfort," the technician informed me. "But stay as still as possible."

No problem. I could handle this. After all, discomfort is what I'd been experiencing for weeks now. But I was totally unprepared for what took place.

"Now again, lie very still. Here we go."

The table I'd been strapped to began revolving, stopping now and then to suspend me upside down in midair. Then it began a rapid spinning movement that created a bursting pain in my ear drums. Somehow I held back a scream and stayed still. I didn't want to move and have to do this again.

On my way home, exhausted and upset, I felt more and more desperate and alone.

"The test indicates inflammation of the inner ear," the doctor informed me the next day. "You have acute labyrinthitis, and that's causing your vertigo and discomfort."

Labrinthitis—inflammation of the inner ear! What a relief to learn I had something, some real disease that they could treat me for! The doctor now had my complete attention. I had needed this reassurance that my illness wasn't psychosomatic, that it wasn't just some kind of emotional problem. Now the doctors would believe me and would be able to help me. At last! Now I can get on with my life; it's going to be all right. The end is in sight . . . or so my thoughts went that day. I listened intently as he explained the disease and treatment.

"In simple terms, vertigo is a sickening feeling of dizziness," he concluded.

"That's a good description," I said. "And I'm so weak it's hard to hold my body up. How did this happen?"

"Probably the result of a viral infection," he said. "It could also account for your present fatigue."

"What can you do for it?" I asked. "How long will it last?"

"Every case is different," he said. Then he told me about an experiment where large doses of Valium had been found to be an effective treatment for this type of vertigo.

"Would you try that?" he asked. "Perhaps it will help you."

I felt so ill that I was willing to try anything. I was actually happy they had finally found something. But that would be my secret—I wasn't about to tell anyone that I was glad I was really sick. Glad at least that it wasn't all in my imagination. I was giddy with delight. I had labyrinthitis! Acute, no less! Wonder where they got that word. Nothing cute about something acute. Beverly, you're no comedienne, that's for sure. Tell your head to shut up, just for a few minutes. What did the doctor say? Something about a mild decrease of hearing in my right ear. Nuts! My right ear is fine. It's just too busy listening to my head.

That day I started the Valium therapy.

All during my illness, Glen had been wonderful. No man had been that good to me. I admired and respected him. Again and again I asked myself—was this love?

One day Glen and I were sitting on my lanai watching the sun set. We were both very quiet, and he took my hand. "I love you," he whispered.

I saw the tears in his eyes as he leaned over to kiss me. An overwhelming need for him swept through my body. This must be love, I thought. I felt relaxed and secure, knowing that we would have a whole lifetime together.

Glen and I talked of marriage, of our future together, and the next few weeks were happy ones for me. I wanted this bliss to last forever. Too soon I would learn that nothing lasts forever.

But for the moment I was encouraged by my improvement. The Valium seemed to help, and I was still taking it. Then one day the sick feeling returned in full force. Oh, no! I panicked. Tests again, and more tests.

When I wasn't undergoing medical tests, I stayed in bed a great deal. At least the Valium helped me sleep, but rest at the apartment was not like rest at the hospital. Glen and I began to get on each other's nerves. The physical pain was getting to me, too, and I started drinking to try to get some relief.

The dizziness, along with my other symptoms, persisted. Weakness and fatigue were the worst. Pain and confusion ran a close second, and the low-grade fever had never completely gone away. I was rapidly losing weight and was now twenty-five pounds below normal. I had always been active and full of energy, so this sudden weakness puzzled me as much as it did the doctors. My days were spent seeing specialists and going from lab to lab for testing. Every suspected disease was either treated or ruled out.

This was to be the pattern of my life for many years to come. In the next year alone, I saw nearly thirty specialists.

I was so tired, and it was not an ordinary fatigue. I was not listless but lifeless. The pain increased and my confusion deepened. I was having nightly fights with Glen, and they were more than I could handle.

When I had first become ill, I had thought Glen a treasure. He seemed to really want to take care of me. But couldn't I take care of myself, I wondered. Why did he think I couldn't? Was he trying to control me? I shuddered, and then I remembered how nice it was to have someone who cared. But now we were having trouble.

I became very nervous from all the testing and not

knowing what was wrong with me. The doctors could not find any organic reason for my deteriorating physical condition, and as my pain and confusion grew, so did my need for drugs. Physically I ached all over, and in spite of the tremendous weight loss, my body felt huge and full of pressure, as if there were some horrible force pushing from within. The pain was unbearable. My body felt as if it were being torn apart, so I returned to Dr. Woodbury to see if he could help me.

But one thing I wasn't going to do was let him see me cry. These days I was continually on the verge of crying; tears were always there, just below the surface. Sometimes, in the loneliness of my living room, with drink in hand, I was able to let them flow. But I never, never cried in front of my doctor. And I felt a lot of conflict about breaking down in front of Glen, too.

"Don't cry," I had heard as a child when I'd fall down. "It doesn't hurt."

I recalled that it did hurt, but wild horses couldn't have dragged that out of me. I was shy and sensitive; but even when my feelings were hurt, I never let it show. Five years old or forty-five—I would not reveal my pain. As a child, I worried that my parents might not love me if I cried or complained, and I carried this fear into adulthood, relating it to other people as well. It seemed to me that I had to keep doing things to win love and approval, but no matter how hard I tried or what I did, I never felt loved.

It was important not to show my feelings to strangers either. And this doctor was most certainly a stranger to me. They all were. In fact, the more doctors I saw, the stranger they became.

Again the Valium dosage was increased to relax my muscle spasms. "I don't know how you're walking around with that much Valium," the doctor said. "I wouldn't be able to stand up."

Actually, I wasn't standing up too well, nor was I

walking too well. I simply put one foot in front of the other and floated. But I wasn't going to tell him that! Besides, as I was to learn years later, at that time I had a very high tolerance to drugs. The Valium didn't affect me then as much as it would most people, and as I continued taking it I had to increase the dosage to even feel its effect at all.

During the next year I had repeated attacks of so-called "flu," with severe stomach pains. Twice I was rushed to the hospital for suspected ruptured appendix.

There were many days I could not move out of bed. I lost my job and lived on disability insurance. All the stabilizing routines of my life disappeared, and I felt as if I wasn't any good to anyone. The low-grade fevers, blurry vision and vertigo continued, and infections that lasted for weeks were as baffling as the disabling fatigue that ruled my life. I didn't know what could be wrong with me!

Not able to function either physically or emotionally, I felt as if I were in an invisible cage. In addition to being weak, I had begun to feel disoriented, with a sensation of being disconnected from the world and the people around me. It was as if I were watching everyone from a distance. The rest of the world was moving, walking, talking; I was standing still in my cage screaming for help, but it was a silent scream. No one could hear me.

My emotional state worsened, I became convinced that I was losing my mind. Why couldn't anyone help me, I wondered. Without warning, my entire life had been totally disrupted. It would be years before I learned that my symptoms were those of a baffling and little-known disease; I only knew that my thinking was confused and my body was in pain.

"Your vertigo is not severe enough to be causing the discomfort and fatigue you're having," one of the doctors commented impatiently. "This type of fatigue syndrome could be a sign of emotional distress."

There was that knot in my stomach again. Was I going crazy? There just didn't seem to be any reason for an emotional crisis in my life. Some of my years in California had been hectic, certainly not total bliss, but I had survived the bad experiences and treasured the good ones.

In my first marriage, we had three beautiful healthy children, my dream come true. I also taught school, another childhood dream. But, over the years, I took on too much, pushed myself too hard. I was an overdoer, a workaholic, always moving at top speed, even though there were times that I felt extraordinary fatigue. This fatigue had troubled me as a child, but it worsened as I became an adult. It seemed that the older I got, the less endurance I had and the harder I strived.

However, it wasn't until my second marriage that my health took a real downhill turn. My bouts with fatigue got longer and more frequent, along with numerous episodes of flu symptoms. So, plagued by exhaustion, I let my work and my home life suffer. I attributed it all to my workload and an unfortunate marriage.

The children and I were survivors, and we made it through a second divorce. I left teaching to go into secretarial work, and the years passed quickly as my children grew to young adulthood, and one by one moved away from home to attend the university.

One year my girlfriend suggested that we take a trip to Hawaii. At that time I knew little about the Islands, but her idea sounded like fun. Both of us were the impulsive type, so within a few days we found ourselves on the enchanting island of Oahu, driving to Waikiki.

I fell in love with the Islands, and I immediately

knew that this was where I wanted to live. Los Angeles had become smoggy and congested, and for years I had been thinking of moving, longing for a simpler life. Now was my chance.

Even though I wanted a less complicated way of life, I was still a "city" girl, so I chose the Island of Oahu. There I could work in downtown Honolulu and live in Waikiki. I would have the best of two worlds: the beauty and simplicity of the Islands and the excitement of Waikiki! I approached this adventurous move feeling strong, healthy and confident. There had been no recent episodes of illness, the trauma of my second divorce had long been over, and my three children were doing well on their own.

As the months passed, I did not regret the move. I lived in the midst of untold beauty, and my passion for the Islands increased. Although I missed my children, I was an attractive woman, enjoying life and happy with my work when this illness began.

Now, a malady that no doctor could identify had changed everything. I was no longer able to think, and my body seemed to have a separate mind controlling its movements. I was becoming desperate. I felt appallingly ill, but I wondered if the doctors believed me. By now, it seemed they were all convinced that it was an emotional problem.

2
Prescription Drug Addiction

The pain in my joints and weakness throughout my body was unpredictable, coming and going with disturbing irregularity. And it wandered around in my body, first in one part and then another, changing its location every few days. I became certain that this couldn't be an ordinary, run-of-the-mill kind of pain. It had to be psychosomatic.

According to teachings of long ago that repeated themselves over and over in my head like a broken record, and according to my doctors, this was emotionally-caused pain. I was worn out by months of going from doctor to doctor, countless tests, the doctors' looks, and no diagnosis. Terribly frightened of this unknown thing that was happening to me, I seemed to be sinking deeper and deeper into the abyss of pain that controlled my body and my life. Inwardly I also felt anger at myself for continuing to consult the medical profession. Each time I became determined to stop seeing doctors, a new pain or symptom would develop somewhere in my body, and I would think that this time the doctors would surely be able to help me. My head said, "You will die from this if you don't get medical attention." So off I would march to another doctor. My life was a living hell. I had no energy.

I isolated myself from people, from my friends, even from Marilyn, using excuse after excuse. I remembered how kind she was, her concern for me that day six months ago when I'd had to suddenly leave the beach and go home. "Just a little tired today and I feel a little dizzy, that's all." If only that had been all! How could I have foreseen the seemingly endless torment that would follow that day? I used to love spending time with Marilyn. She was easy to talk to, easy to be yourself with. It was difficult, almost impossible, to feel any way but happy around her contagious laugh. Now I couldn't stand to be with anyone except Glen, who, in spite of our frequent quarrels, was my constant evening companion.

My coordination was so poor that it embarrassed me to eat with anyone. I never knew if my hand would be steady enough to transport food from the plate to my mouth. I was in a constant panic, convinced that I was losing my mind. My condition reached the point where it was no longer advisable for me to live alone. I loved Glen and being with him was a great source of comfort to me. Yet it was not enough to overcome the fear of marriage. Glen got a marriage license and I got sicker.

I didn't tell my family or mainland friends that I was sick. When they visited, I took my pills, put on a happy face and acted as well as I could. I didn't want to worry them. California was a long way off, and I didn't think it would do anyone any good to know that I was ill. One time, on my parents' fiftieth wedding anniversary, I planned a trip to California to celebrate this special occasion with them. But I was too ill for the trip. I told my family that I had a bad ear infection. That was not too far from the truth as far as it went.

Since I had canceled my flight, Mom and Dad took a second honeymoon to visit me and the Islands. I kept the truth about my illness a secret.

In order to keep up a pretense of well-being, I took more and more pills. Doctors were now recommending and supplying me with a tranquilizer, a sedative, a stimulant and a pain killer. With the help of these drugs, I forced myself to move at full speed, only to collapse every few days, unable to move at all. Several times I tried returning to work, but the results were always the same—after one day I was unable to hold my body up. I still couldn't tell Glen how really sick I'd been feeling. No man wants to be bothered with someone who is constantly ill, I thought, and I wanted to give our relationship every chance. It never occurred to me that we might get along better if he knew the whole truth and could then understand why I was so moody, so easily upset. Our relationship was clearly going downhill. But then, so was I. In my confused state I thought that maybe our relationship would improve again, that maybe we could get married, if I just didn't tell Glen how ill I was. I panicked at the mention of marriage, but I really loved this man, or so I felt at the time.

I continued to wander from doctor to doctor, lab to lab, hoping to find the answer. I was no longer thinking; my mind was totally confused, and while I had no energy, I seemed compelled to continue this medical merry-go-round. I needed more and more of whatever drug I happened to be taking at the time, but nothing was working. In the daytime, I couldn't relax and I wandered around in a fog. At night, I couldn't sleep without alcohol or my medication, without the drug that kept me in a fog all the following day. My fearful thoughts tumbled over one another, confusing me even more. My condition grew steadily worse and I wanted to die, but some inner force kept me moving. I shouted and prayed for help while attempting to control a situation over which I had no control.

I had no respect for this kind of pain, so I tried to ignore it; and when that became impossible, I would accept sedation rather than having to face yet another skeptical doctor. How could one complain about inconsistent pain that never even stayed in one place, pain that I couldn't even describe? Was I a hypochondriac? Was I becoming a drug addict? No, drug addiction didn't happen to people like me. I pushed the thought out of my mind and took another pill.

The terror became stronger each day. I cleaned the apartment, sweeping and vacuuming to clear the fog in my head created by the pills I took to keep moving. I floated aimlessly from room to room, singing, "I'm looking for me, where can I be? Jumping around, can't find the ground. I'm looking for me. Behind the door, under the bed, under the pillows where he laid his head. Where can I be? I'm looking for me." And then I'd burst into uncontrollable tears. What had happened to the real Beverly? I wasn't her anymore; I was someone else, and I didn't know who. I wanted to be able to laugh again.

One morning, after a particularly restless night, I felt dizzier than usual. I wandered around the apartment and finally collapsed my now bony body onto the couch. I hated the confusion in my head. I had to get outside to some fresh air. Fresh air, that's it, I thought. I grabbed my keys and walked unsteadily out the door and down six flights of stairs, clinging to the railing, afraid to wait for the elevator. (Someone might see me in this condition.) Once outside, I carefully made my way down the three short blocks to Kalakaua Avenue, Waikiki's main street. I wanted to be around people. I wanted to see the ocean. I didn't walk, I floated down Kalakaua Avenue praying no one would notice me. My equilibrium was off and my feet seemed to be walking six inches above the ground. I felt drunk, even though I hadn't yet had a drink. Then I saw my friend Darlene walking toward me.

"Bev! Hi. Where are you off to?" she said as we almost knocked each other over.

Darn, she'll notice how I'm feeling. I smiled. We talked and laughed, and for the first few minutes I was genuinely happy to see her. But I knew that I had to get away, fast. I was getting dizzier every second and was terrified that I would pass out if I stood there any longer.

"Let's get together soon," I said in a flurry. "Have to dash now, really good to see you. I'll call next week."

We hugged and I hurried away, leaving Darlene with a bewildered look on her face, and my mind traveling faster than I. I have to get home, I thought. I can't stand up. It's these pills. I'll never take another pill. I'm getting confused from all these pills. No more! I rushed home and collected the medicine bottles from around my apartment, twenty-six in all, and threw them in the drawer of my dresser and slammed it shut. I thought of tossing them down the toilet, but I didn't. Later I would regret that.

In June of 1975, Dr. Dailey, the latest in a seemingly endless line of doctors, referred me to Dr. Logan, a psychiatrist. I was nervous but willing to see this new doctor. I desperately wanted to prove to these doctors that there was a physical reason for my fatigue and pain. I would take any kind of test. My mind was all right; it was by body that wasn't working, and the pain was driving me crazy. Oops, careful with that word, someone will lock you up! These were my thoughts as I sat in the psychiatrist's office marking a questionaire that seemed to be preoccupied with my physical complaints, rather than my feelings.

The questions were endless—had I ever had bladder problems, muscle weakness, back pain, headaches? Sure, I've had those problems, but I don't have them today. How should I answer? I don't want them to think I'm a hypochondriac. Let's see, when I had my back surgery—no, that was over fifteen years ago. Still . . . so much for being honest. I know how to answer this test, I know what they're looking for. There's that same question again, worded in a different way. What a trick, almost caught me on that one. Damn, this test is just a bunch of tricks, and long! My hand and neck are beginning to bother me. Oh! There, they asked that question, too. Can't hold this pen to mark the answers. Who cares, anyway? No one's going to understand. How can I describe what my body's feeling? Or is it my mind? A coldness went through me. A chill, or was it fear? I wiped away the lonely tear that had begun to slide down my cheek.

Dr. Logan's diagnosis was "depressive neurosis, severe." This label was to follow me through many bouts of illness.

I told Dr. Logan that the Valium helped. "It's the only pill that seems to ease the pain and not make me sleepy." So he gave me a prescription for more Valium. Now I was getting it from two doctors. Somewhere in the dark mazes of my mind, I began to be afraid of Valium addiction. I wanted to stop taking it. "Why?" I screamed into the air. "Why do I have to be sick? Why can't they find out what's wrong!"

My parents were shining examples of good health. My father was a pharmacist, and at an early age I had heard about the pitfalls of medication and junk food. I was a child who rarely ate candy or drank soda pop, even though both were always available at my dad's drugstore. I could have had as much as I wanted, but I grew up just knowing that sweets were bad for my teeth, that junk food was detrimental to my health, and the overuse of drugs could be harmful. My sister and I were probably the only two people in the world who preferred a polio shot to the cubes of sugar they started using; to this day I feel guilty if I have a candy bar. I didn't fall for junk food, candy or soda pop, but I became addicted to drugs, supplied by a neat small piece of paper called a prescription.

It was several months before I told Dr. Logan of my fear of addiction. The good doctor promptly took me off Valium and prescribed Thorazine instead, an even stronger tranquilizer. Let me tell you about my reaction to Thorazine, the miracle drug, which I later discovered is used on a regular basis in mental hospitals to keep the patients under control so they won't give the doctors any trouble.

After I took the Thorazine, my body would not respond to my commands. It was as though every time I tried to move in one direction, my body forcefully fought to go the other way. My muscles became spastic and I couldn't hold things in my hands. I went into a semi-hypnotic state. My thinking had been confused before, but now it was totally chaotic. I wandered around the apartment, not knowing where I was.

At ten o'clock the next morning I saw the psychiatrist again. In his office I lay on the floor in a fetal position, with my legs curled up. I couldn't control my actions.

"Do you see what you're doing?" Dr. Logan said.

Of course, dummy, I thought, I just can't help myself. That's why I'm here. You're the doctor, why don't you help me?

But out loud I said, "Sorry, guess I lost control." I got up slowly and awkwardly from the floor. I told him about the disorientation I experienced since taking the Thorazine. He gave me a large injection of Valium in order to counteract the Thorazine, and then led me out into the hall.

"Wait in here," he said, motioning me into the room next to his office. It was tiny, with no windows, a small couch against one wall, a table against another. I paced back and forth for what seemed like hours. I was exhausted. How long was I supposed to wait? What time was it? How many hours did he want me to stay here? There was an unearthly quietness about the room.

After what seemed an eternity, my body stopped twitching and I began to calm down. This is more like it, I reflected. Now I'm relaxed. I sighed with relief. I sat on the couch waiting for someone to come and tell me what to do next. I was calm. I was all right now. The doctor would surely be pleased.

After a while, I lay down and dropped off to sleep. I dreamt of huge men chasing me, their arms outstretched, grabbing at me, but always missing. At the last instant, just before their arms would engulf me, I'd run a little faster and escape. Then I was on my knees, crawling, in the middle of a vast desert. The men had disappeared. I was moving along the sand trying to reach something. What was it? Soon I was almost immobile. I kept trying to move faster, faster, but my body was too heavy, the pain was too great . . . I couldn't. Try—faster, faster, I must get there.

I awoke on the couch, grateful to be away from the dream, my body covered with perspiration.

Why hadn't anyone come to get me? I walked over to the door and opened it a crack, listening for movement or voices outside, from the other offices. There wasn't a sound. Quickly I shut the door. Should I leave? No, he said to wait.

The Valium was wearing off, and I began pacing up and down again. I couldn't stop moving. The floor seemed closer, and my mind was reeling. Why had he left me alone? Where was everybody? Why didn't someone come and tell me I could leave? The tears fought to emerge but, even though I was alone, I held them back. No point in becoming hysterical, I thought, with panic building up inside me, then they'll really think I'm crazy. They might lock me up. I certainly didn't want them to think anything was wrong with my mind!

I continued to move around the room, which

seemed to be getting tinier and more confining the longer I was there. What time was it? How late did the office stay open? Again, I opened the door—very hesitantly—and walked on tip-toe through the dark hallway. "Hello," I whispered, peering through each office doorway. "Anyone here?" The rooms were all empty. They had left me alone. My doctor—everyone—had completely forgotten about me. The tears finally came as I walked through the waiting room, into the building lobby and then ran out to the street. It was seven o'clock. I'd been there all day.

Soon after the Thorazine incident I began having muscle spasms in my back and neck, and severe joint pain, especially in the mornings and evenings. I was also having urinary and heart problems. More specialists were consulted.

On June 12, 1975, I was admitted to another hospital. A complete blood workup was done, or so I thought. As usual, nothing abnormal was found. Then an orthopedic surgeon was called.

"I had back surgery, a laminectomy, about ten years ago," I told him. "The pain and spasms feel the same as before that surgery, only this time it's in my neck and down my arm."

X-rays were taken. The next day, the doctor sat calmly on the edge of my bed. "You have bone spurs and degenerative arthritis in the cervical area," he said. "Although this sort of cervical problem can cause pain and fatigue, I can find no organic reason for such extreme difficulties as you're experiencing."

I was given an anti-inflammatory drug along with two other medications. I left the hospital with prescriptions for Valium, the anti-inflammatory drug Motrin, and Darvocet N for pain.

For years prior to this illness, I had crusaded against drugs; now I was under the care of three doctors and taking twenty-six pills daily. I had entered the nightmarish world of prescription drugs and still did not have a diagnosis. My medicine chest looked like a pharmacy. I had pills to relax my muscles, for pain, for inflammation, for sleep and to pep me up. I had so many recurring infections, some lasting for months, that I was repeatedly on antibiotics. And each new antibiotic seemed to set off a secondary infection elsewhere in my body. Worst of all was the stark terror and despair that I felt inside. My weight had dropped from 135 to 100 pounds. I was afraid that I was dying, and at the same time, I prayed that I would.

For the next eighteen months, despite psychiatric counseling and a daily usage of Valium, my many symptoms persisted. Different ones came and went with disturbing irregularity. I was dizzy most of the time, and my eyes wouldn't focus. Fatigue devastated me. It was almost too much of an effort just to breathe.

As my pain and confusion increased, so did my craving for drugs. The Valium that I had grown to love as a friend was controlling my life. But the pills were not working fast enough for me, so I turned to alcohol again. Before long I began drinking and using medication on a daily basis, alternating between the two until soon I was using the alcohol to swallow my pills. This combination should have killed me, but by some miracle my life, such as it was, went on. I was locked in my invisible cage, and the walls were getting smaller and smaller. My inner screams were like miniature bombs exploding throughout my body and mind. I didn't know how to verbalize my need for help, and I kept telling myself that I should be able to handle my own problems. Yet every day I was faced with the emotional anguish of not knowing what was wrong with me.

I finally decided that it must be the pills and alcohol that were causing my confusion. I stopped drinking and I stopped taking the sleeping pills. I needed the other medications, I kept telling myself, I could not get through a day without them.

After going without sleep for three days, I happened to see a TV advertisement for an over-the-counter sleep medication. I broke into a grin. At last, a safe way of getting some sleep! I rushed to the nearest drug store.

I found the wonder pills right away and handed them to the clerk. "For a friend," I said, giving her my brightest smile. I laughed nervously trying to cover up a twinge of guilt, then continued with my pretense. "She's been having some problems and has a little trouble sleeping. Do you think these will help?"

"Sure," she answered. "I take them all the time. Work great."

"Oh good," I said. "They're not dangerous, are they? I mean, like addictive or anything?"

"Heavens no! They're perfectly safe. We couldn't sell them without a prescription if they weren't."

What a relief. This was not a drug, yet I would get some sleep.

That night I slept peacefully and woke up the next morning feeling relaxed and happy. I hadn't needed any prescriptions for drugs, just a little night aid that everyone took.

By afternoon, I was shaking as I walked into my favorite restaurant for lunch. "Hi, Bev," the waitress said. "Hey you look beat. How about a martini?"

I hesitated. I wanted to quit, but surely one little drink wouldn't hurt, and I needed something to calm me down. Maybe those pills I took last night hadn't been such a good idea. No, the clerk had said they were all right to take; I just needed more sleep.

"Good idea," I smiled. "I haven't been getting enough sleep lately. I feel edgy and a martini might help."

By evening I was back to drinking and using sleeping pills. Soon Glen and I were both drinking excessively.

Weeks passed. The more my body hurt, the more my relationship with Glen deteriorated. I became increasingly discontented. I couldn't marry anybody while I felt like this. Glen and I broke up and six months later he married. I never saw him again, but I was too muddled to care.

Throughout all my illnesses a most frustrating fact was that I didn't look sick, even during the times that I felt deathly ill.

"Bev, you look so well, you can't be sick." This was my doctors' and my friends' constant cry. It seemed to me that everyone thought I was a hypochondriac, and I was tired of their insinuations. I decided to pretend that I felt as well as I looked and no longer tell anyone of this daily pain that I couldn't even describe anyway. I would sedate myself and ignore the pain.

Every day I wrote about my anguish and despair, and then set to work cleaning my apartment. I worked as hard as I could, but the pain only got worse, and I became more confused than ever.

"My body's moving faster and faster," I wrote. "I can't stop. Or is it my head that won't stop? I hurt all over, but I can't stop moving. I keep cooking, cleaning, eating, drinking. Please, dear God, help me to stop. I'm so tired."

My many illnesses continued. Mostly the doctors treated the inflammation and pain that came and went throughout my body, shattering it at irregular intervals. I was exhausted. I felt as if I were carrying a thousand pounds, and every movement was an effort.

The apartment I lived in was on the twenty-second floor. There were times, mostly at night, when I wondered how I managed to keep from going over the edge of the lanai and ending it all. With my mind exploding and my body collapsing, I screamed to God for help. There had to be some way out of this nightmare. Again I resolved to ignore the pain and never, never see another doctor or take another test. If I were going to die, I would do it alone and not subject myself to any more humiliation, to any more of the doctors' pathetic looks and angry words.

On February 12, 1977, I stood unsteadily in front of my dressing table, counting the blurry maze of prescription bottles. Somewhere in the inner depths of what sanity I had left, I knew that I had to break out of this vicious cycle—pain, drugs and confusion, ad infinitum. I flushed all the pills down the toilet—finally—and poured the alcohol into the sink.

"I must do this," I screamed aloud. I was too muddled to call anyone, telling myself that I should be able to handle my own problems.

For five days I hallucinated alone in my apartment. Dreaming or waking, my visions were terrifying, horrible. The worst came during full moon, its light shining brightly through my bedroom window. I saw insects crawling everywhere. They were there on the bed, the walls, the floors. They crept along the nerve endings in my body, under my skin and on top. I itched all over. Then I watched them grow in size, the small black bugs getting larger and larger. I cringed in terror as one crawled along the pillow toward my face. Somehow I knew they weren't really there, but I couldn't stop the fear that engulfed me. As if the bugs were not enough, I began to hear hideous screams coming from somewhere. Suddenly I realized that they were coming from me! Involuntary screams that started deep inside, welled slowly up to my throat, then escaped my lips.

I continued to scream. My mouth was open and the sound emerging from it was one loud wail, over which

I had no control. I lay there and stared in horror as the forms jumped from the pillow onto my hand and moved slowly up my arm. I batted and struck at them, but the nothings wouldn't leave. I had to get away. I forced my fingers to reach up and turn the light on. The bugs disappeared. The noise stopped. But for a long time I was too terrified to sleep.

When I finally did sleep, I would awaken a few hours later in a cold sweat, paralyzed with fear. My muscles were twitching almost constantly, day and night, and my body felt as though it were being torn apart. My insides were on fire. I paced from room to room, totally disoriented. I tried to cling to a reality that seemed so far away that I couldn't quite reach it. However, somehow, an inner strength, greater than my own, kept me going. I knew it was that strength that had seen me through so far, keeping me alive, barely alive. Finally, after six days of little sleep and even less food, I gave way to total panic and phoned my psychiatrist. He was angry that I had stopped taking the drugs so abruptly! "Cold turkey," he called it. "That was a very foolish and dangerous thing to do."

So, on February 17, 1977, with my mind submerged in a deep fog, I succumbed to my first hospitalization for drug withdrawal.

3
Diagnosis of Lupus

The minute the door clanged shut behind me, I knew this was no regular hospital. My mind pushed deeper into panic—I had to get out of here! A nurse took me to my room, and we walked down a long corridor, marked with arrows and lines painted on the floor, to a locked door. It opened, then closed—with me on the other side. My head cleared. I had to do something, anything, to get away from this place, as fast as I could. In that instant, I was so filled with fear that I forgot I was there voluntarily, to get help.

I continued my game of pretending to be okay, except when talking with Dr. Logan, my psychiatrist. With others, I had to keep up a front of well-being, only then would I win their love and approval. Who were these "others"? Anyone and everyone. I wanted to please the world!

In the hospital, I fought to keep my mind active. I organized exercise classes, swam in the hospital pool until my limbs ached, and I never complained. I just wanted to get out of this crazy place. Normally a shy person, I talked and joked incessantly with anyone who would respond, inmates or staff. The laughter kept my mind alive, helped keep me sane. Around me, people were screaming, walking up and down the halls talking to themselves, living in worlds of their own. My terror grew worse at night when I would be awakened by another patient's outcry, or found one standing by my bed staring down at me.

I would not cooperate with Dr. Logan. He was trying to feed me medicine—poison, I thought—to keep me from functioning. I considered him my enemy, and maybe he was. I told him I needed help and would do anything he wanted, but I couldn't. He wanted me to wear a hospital gown and be an invalid, totally dependent on him, but I wouldn't do it. I refused, telling him I would wear my own clothes.

In a weak moment, I allowed Dr. Logan to give me Thorazine. I didn't even ask what the medication was until, once again, the spastic symptoms appeared. The staff members became concerned and called the doctor immediately. The medication was stopped.

Several days before leaving the hospital, I made arrangements to go into an addiction treatment facility. On March 14, after three and a half weeks in a mental hospital, I entered the 24-hour program.

Our day began at 6 a.m. There wasn't much time for writing, but I kept in constant touch with my family because I didn't want them to worry. However, except for my sister, I never told any of them about my illnesses or where I now lived, and I wasn't totally honest with her, either. She would have been worried out of her mind if she'd known the kind of place this really was. I was trying to help myself, and something told me I couldn't make it at my apartment alone, so I had fought to get into this facility. Who would want to be here anyway, I sometimes wondered. My companions were parolees, thieves and murderers, as well as the plain, everyday varieties of addicts and alcoholics, like me. Many were there as the only alternative to prison. If they left—that is, escaped—the staff called the police. When they were caught they would be returned to prison, not the facility.

But all of us had one thing in common: we were

withdrawing from one form or another of drugs, trying to find a way to live without them. I needed help to find a way to cope with the pain in my body and my mind without using the pills that were destroying me.

I hoped that this program would help me, and I really worked at it. I was so sick and tired of being sick and tired that I was willing to do anything, but I didn't know how to be honest.

The facility was like an unreal city. At first I was afraid of everyone, then I fell victim to their likable qualities and expected more from them than they could deliver. I wanted honest and loving friendships, but I couldn't really trust or confide in anyone. Whatever I said to individuals would be repeated to the group. It may have been part of the treatment, but to me it was another sign that my new friends were unpredictable. However, in the five months, no one ever got hurt there, and nothing was ever stolen. It was uncanny. In some ways, we were bound together and protected each other. I didn't realize that we weren't working with a full deck—any of us. In fact, my awareness of anything at all was at a very low ebb. We were all going through drug withdrawal, and it was like becoming a child again, with raw emotions, dependent on the authority in charge. None of us liked that and we took our rebellion out on each other with verbal abuse.

I never tried to leave, even though the doors were always open, and even though unhappiness permeated my existence there. I started complaining on a daily basis; we all did, about everyone and everything. Hostility reigned—with us, it was the family that flays together stays together. If anyone prayed, I wasn't aware of it. I certainly didn't. On the other side of the coin, there was the laughter and the companionship, the volleyball games and the working together, the tears and the empathy we occasionally gave each other. But always, overshadowing it all, there was the loneliness, the utter loneliness. Even in the midst of all these people, I felt it. I also had lost my valued privacy, but worst of all was the deep-rooted anger that I felt but didn't know how to release.

I was being controlled by fear, although I never understood what I was so afraid of. I thought it was fear of being on my own, alone with my cloudy mind. At least here I am taken care of, I thought, no decisions to make because people told me what to do and when to do it. I hated it! But my day, bad as it was, was structured, and I could no longer do that myself. So I stayed. If I left, I knew I would not be allowed to come back.

Of the sixty people living there, only six were women. It was not a place for the "softer" sex, and they were screened very carefully. Most women wouldn't—and didn't—want to be there. The physical work was too hard, the pressure too great, and the restrictions too heavy. I had trouble getting in. When my application was rejected, I became even more determined to enter this program. The staff didn't believe that I could take the group confrontations, but I was stronger than they thought. People had always been deceived by my quiet nature.

My persistence paid off and I talked my way in. But could I stay? Could I take the pressure without cracking up completely? I had to try.

We all shared in the work; cleaning, cooking, and working out in the yard. Then there were the classes and therapy groups that went on all day, but the nights were long and empty. When I first arrived, I didn't walk in—I was still floating from drug withdrawals. My feet never felt as if they were touching the ground. I was very ill. For the first several weeks—or was it months?—I was afraid to sleep. The nights and my nightmares were ghastly, but I could take it, or so

I tried to convey. Inside, I was wilting away.

I constantly dreamt that I was being buried alive. The coffin was open, but I couldn't move. When the lid closed, I'd wake up terrified. So instead of going back to sleep, I walked in the hall all night, talking to the other walkers. Our bodies kept moving and we couldn't sleep—we couldn't even relax. We were too used to having drugs to do that for us. I later learned that one young man I'd spent many a night talking to jumped off the roof of an apartment building two months after I left the facility. Another died in an automobile accident, drunk, trapped in the flames of his own car.

I enrolled in a psychology class, via the radio. I would become a counselor; helping others was the answer. Speak of the blind leading the blind! I deluded myself and others. In a letter to my sister, I wrote of this fantastic opportunity as if that were why I was there. I had convinced myself that this was what I needed to do to get well. This had to be the answer to the dreadful weakness and fatigue that was still with me. So I lied to my family and to myself, to cover up the embarrassment of my life.

Then I started brooding. What was I doing in this place anyway? I didn't belong here; there was nothing wrong with me. I'm well . . . and so my thinking went. Immediately my mind devised plans of escape, escape from a place that I had come to voluntarily, escape from a place I could leave anytime I chose. Still I stayed. So much for my rational thinking.

Despite the emotional ups and downs, life there was boring, tedious and filled with hard work. Nonetheless, I remained for five months, all the while complaining, criticizing and literally despising the facility I had pushed so hard to get into. I knew, I just knew, that this was where I needed to be, but I never reached the point of being comfortable, and the lack of freedom got to me more and more.

Time had no meaning for me. Each 24-hour period was emotionally torturous, but somehow the months did pass, and I did make progress. I started feeling better, more human. Then one day I woke up unable to move my head. It was September, 1977. I was having severe spasms in my neck and there was a tingling sensation radiating down my left arm. My hand and fingers were numb. I managed to get up and didn't tell anyone until the pain became too intense for me to work. I was excused from the daily activities and sent to a hospital for x-rays.

"Your arthritis is worse," the doctor said. "Your joints are inflamed and there are bone spurs in the cervical area of your spine." This was nothing new. I was given Motrin to reduce the inflammation, and Darvocet N-100 was prescribed for pain.

I now had a choice of remaining at the addiction treatment facility without using the drugs prescribed, or leaving. In addition to the severe pain, nerve damage was a possibility if my condition was left untreated. I chose to leave, but wondered if I was heading right back where I had started five months earlier.

I took the medication and became as spaced out as I had been with the Valium. Then I was hospitalized for cervical traction and physical therapy. After ten days, surgery was suggested to remove the bone spurs. That would alleviate the pressure on the cervical nerves, I had been told several times. I decided against the surgery, and on Thanksgiving Day of 1977 I moved to California to be closer to my family. I would seek medical consultation there.

Once in California, a university medical center seemed the logical place to go. I'd had spinal surgery at one of these centers fifteen years earlier, and I had great confidence in them. Once you went through their medical department, you got a precise and complete diagnosis. Certain that they'd find all my problems, I sat patiently in the waiting room. Six hours later, I didn't feel so sure.

Finally, the neurosurgeon examined me. I briefly related my history, being sure to tell her about my experiences with drugs. X-rays were taken and the diagnosis of bone spurs and arthritis in the cervical area was again confirmed.

"None of this is severe enough to cause the pain and fatigue you're having," the doctor said. Her tone and words were very familiar. "Rest at home and come back in two weeks, if you're still having problems." I was given more prescriptions for Valium and Darvocet N-100. Visions of Honolulu crossed my mind. I was too tired to argue, but I didn't fill the prescriptions.

After the six-hour wait and two-hour examination, I barely made it back to my motel. Later I debated about going to the drugstore for the medicines, but the horror of going through another drug withdrawal was stronger than any physical pain I was having.

The following day I awakened with a stiff neck and pain again radiating down my left arm. I went to visit friends, to take my mind off the pain.

"My neck is really hurting," I said, while my girlfriend listened sympathetically. "I can't handle much more of this." I told her what the doctors said. "Honestly, it's that I'm so tired, that's what bothers me the most. I'm so weak, it's an effort to move at all."

"Why don't you take something for the pain," she suggested. "Let's go see Warren. Maybe he can help you." Warren was an old friend who also happened to be a doctor. I hadn't seen him since long before I moved to Hawaii.

Warren gave me some Darvon to relieve the pain. This time I took it. It would be all right; he not only was a doctor, but my friend.

Two days later, I began hallucinating again. The

giant bugs were back. I was in such a confused state of mind I could not make it from the bed to the kitchen and still remember what I had gone into the kitchen for.

Somewhere in the back of my mind, I became deathly afraid of drinking again, so I entered what I prayed would be my last alcohol and drug withdrawal program. This was a facility for women, smaller than the one in Honolulu. For the thirty days that I was there, I again felt the loss of freedom, but this time in a much more loving atmosphere. With the help of newfound friends, I began to find a new way to live without drugs.

The next two years were emotionally and physically painful, but I had been given hope and a faith in the future by people who understood what I was feeling. They had been to similar depths of destruction with alcohol and drugs and had found a solution. Still, with all this, the weakness, fatigue and countless infections persisted. I stayed away from doctors as much as possible. I decided to remain in California for a year to see if being with family, and among new friends, would benefit my physical condition and stop my emotional upheaval. It seemed to me that at last I really belonged somewhere. Strange, that somewhere was California, the very place I had left to move to Hawaii.

Positive changes began to take place within me, and my life gradually became less difficult. I missed the tropical sun of Hawaii, but I felt better in a cooler climate. I missed my friends on the Island, too, but then I had made new ones here. My life was getting better. I remember walking barefoot in the sand along the beach, a warm breeze tugging at me as I watched the waves move in and out. I was grateful for the many blessings in my life. Stronger than ever was my determination to never, never see another doctor.

This resolution, like so many, was short-lived.

In the months that followed, the new inner peace that I had found was marred by the unpredictable weakness and fatigue that continued to plague me. Along with the pain in my joints came a return of the vertigo that had started in Hawaii four years earlier. I had thought drugs had caused this, but here I was, two years off drugs, and my physical problems were the same. Adapt, I thought, but how can I? I'm only fifty years old and my body feels like eighty. My parents have more energy than I have! How do I adapt to that?

My limitations frustrated and depressed me. And again, I had infections that lasted for months and were as bewildering as the disabling fatigue. With each recurring infection, I would go back on medication, and then go through a drug withdrawal period.

I was anxious to get back to a structured and fulfilling life. The only identities I had ever known were that of wife, mother and employee. I was no longer a wife, my children were grown, and I had not been able to work for almost five years. I took a two-week temporary job, but after just one week, I developed a sore throat and stiff muscles. Antibiotics were prescribed but did nothing to help the stiffness in my muscles.

Then one morning in 1979, the spasms in my neck returned with such force that I was again unable to move my head. I dragged my body slowly into the bathroom. Sharp pains were shooting down my arm and the joints in my fingers were so stiff that I could not hold a toothbrush. "Not again," I mumbled. My hands felt numb. I buried my head in the towel to hold back the tears that started running down my face.

After several weeks, I found myself going to another doctor, one more time. The waiting room was filled with patients. Sitting opposite me was a young man who had been injured in football practice. In a semi-hypnotic state, I watched him as he read the signatures on his cast. Would they put a cast around my neck?

I sat there for an hour, engulfed in pain. Finally it became too much and I slumped on the couch, unable to hold my head up any longer. My purse made a good pillow.

"Just a few more minutes," the nurse said. I waited another hour.

The worst part was the anxiety. Years of going to doctors had made me dread talking to them. My problems had to be emotional, just like all those doctors in Honolulu had said. Why couldn't I overcome this? What was I doing here anyway? Why me? My thoughts raced from self-recrimination to self-pity. I wanted to scream them to that young man who had tired of reading his cast and was now drawing on it.

I clung to the hope that maybe this doctor would be different and could help me. It wasn't just the pain in my neck, it was this interminable weakness and fatigue.

When I finally saw Dr. Kyle I mentioned only my neck problem because I didn't want him to think that I was neurotic. First let's treat the neck. He told me that it was a recurrence of a cervical injury I had been treated for ten years earlier. He recommended "conservative treatment," which meant another hospitalization, with physical therapy and traction.

After two weeks in the hospital and a month in traction at home, my spinal problem greatly improved, though there was still some minor discomfort in my arms, shoulders and neck. When I returned for a checkup, my major complaint was fatigue. I was so tired that it was an effort to talk. I listened with increasing despair to what the doctor told me. The tone of his voice and his words were all too familiar.

"Beverly, you have arthritis and bone spurs in the

cervical area," Dr. Kyle began hurriedly. "However, that isn't any reason for your extreme fatigue and weakness, and I don't understand the reason for the ache in your body. Depression can cause all this. Are you upset about anything?"

"Yes," I answered, trying to control my anger. "I'm upset because I'm tired of being in pain!" My eyes filled with tears, and I squeezed them shut to keep from crying. At all costs, I didn't want to cry.

I was referred to a physical therapist who worked with me twice a week and put me on a home program. My muscles began to strengthen, but the heaviness in my body and the swelling in my joints limited my activities. I continued my exercises at home.

During the next few months, the pain came and went with no apparent pattern. Just as before, years earlier, there were days when I could not move out of bed. Then, as mysteriously as it had appeared, the pain and weakness would be gone, only to reappear a few days later in a different part of my body. I was very tired, yet I couldn't sleep, and my vertigo returned. I looked well, in spite of the insomnia, but I felt seriously ill. Once again I thought I was losing my mind, only this time I had no drugs to blame.

"What is happening?" I screamed into the air. Mornings and evenings were the most painful times, but I was told that this was the pattern with arthritis. Still, somewhere in the back of my mind was this nagging doubt that arthritis, as I understood it, was my only problem. I knew people who had arthritis, but I had never heard any of them mention a heavy feeling throughout their bodies. And what about this fatigue and weakness that immobilized me? It had to be something else, but my determination to discover the truth was giving way. I didn't know where to turn.

I continued with physical therapy, which helped to a degree. However, neither I nor the therapist was satisfied with my progress. He too thought my trouble might be more than the diagnosed arthritis and bone spurs.

"Your muscles are still weak," he said. "Have you ever seen a rheumatologist for your arthritic problem?"

I thought of all the specialists I had seen, but for the life of me, I couldn't remember one being a rheumatologist. I was not sure I even knew what one was.

As if reading my mind, the therapist continued. "You look puzzled," he said with a laugh. "A rheumatologist is a specialist in arthritic disorders. There's a good group right across the street. Lots of my patients use them."

A cold fear gripped me. I would keep up my exercises at home, but I would not go to another doctor.

It was a sunny January morning in 1980, but even before I was fully awake, I could feel the oppressive ache throughout my body. Every movement was painful. The nausea went in huge spasms from my stomach through my chest and stuck in my throat. I could taste the fish that I'd eaten the night before. My legs were like heavy wooden stilts, and it was a tremendous effort to lift one foot in front of the other. I moved in slow motion, making my way to the bathroom to heave in the sink.

As I crawled back to bed, a sick sensation surged through my entire being. The tears that had been welling up in my eyes from the pain overflowed, streaking down my face onto the pillow. My body shook with uncontrollable sobs. It was truly starting again. Two years of struggling with drug withdrawal and here I was, right back to six years ago on the Islands.

I was desperate—there had to be an answer to my nightmarish life. Then I remembered the physical therapist's words. I emptied my purse on the bed and searched through the papers. All this mess! Where was that number the therapist had given me? Maybe in my wallet. Ah, yes, here it is, right where I'd put it, behind last week's grocery receipt. The Arthritis Center. Good name. They should know what they're doing. I made an appointment with a rheumatologist for the following week.

After entering the medical building, I stood outside Dr. Reed's office, praying for a solution that would lead me back to an active, normal life. Not wanting to be disappointed again, I tried not to let my expectations soar. Still, my intuition told me that somewhere behind this door I would find my answer. I would tell this doctor the entire story of my past experiences, even if they did sound psychosomatic. It was the truth, and the doctor needed to know all the facts.

I was very uncomfortable sitting before this new doctor, detailing my complex medical history, my past and present, and listing all my symptoms, but I was determined to be honest. My drug experiences were not easy to talk about, and even worse was having to relate the weird physical happenings. I felt certain that I sounded like a hypochondriac describing my many symptoms and illnesses. The migratory inconsistent pain, chronic weakness and fatigue, weight loss and fevers, stiffness and swelling, flu and viral infections—my list was endless. Would the doctor prejudge and label me a neurotic? I had to chance it.

Dr. Reed asked me many questions. The final one was, "Have you ever had a positive Wassermann test?"

"No," I answered, puzzled and distressed by her inquiry. "Why? Are you suggesting I have syphilis?"

"No," she smiled, "but sometimes a false positive

test for syphilis indicates another disease."

I didn't ask what that might be.

After a thorough examination, blood and urine samples were taken. I was to return for an evaluation of all the tests; in the meantime my medical records would be rounded up. I had brought some with me from Hawaii, the others being scattered among the four doctors in my local area. Forwarding records could be slow. Wanting help quickly, I began collecting the records myself, going from doctor to doctor. This new doctor would have all the information I could get to her as fast as I could bring it. My hopes skyrocketed.

During the next week, as I remembered the doctor's questions, my optimism faltered. I began to feel discouraged, thinking that I might have goofed up my answers to her queries. How could I explain the craziness of this pain that traveled around in my body? Once again I was afraid that the doctor would find nothing organically wrong with me. I worried that again I would be told that I had arthritis, "but arthritis alone is not enough to cause all these problems. Are you upset about something?" I didn't think I could handle that happening again.

Would this doctor really be able to help me? Was she taking me seriously? These thoughts tormented me all week, but I pushed on, getting my medical files, and taking each one to the doctor's office as I collected it. Her receptionist expressed surprise, but I wasn't going to waste any more time. I had to know, one way or the other. Either this doctor could help me or she couldn't. There was no middle of the road here. And she needed all my records to make a diagnosis.

By the time I again entered the doctor's office I felt tired and depressed. I fully expected to hear the "it's all in your head" routine, though deep down I prayed that she would be able to help me. And as soon as I looked at her, I knew that this time was indeed going to be different.

"Your blood tests indicate lupus," she said. There was warmth and understanding in her voice—and was that compassion? Well, *I* didn't understand. I was dumfounded!

"What is lupus?" I finally managed to ask. Did I have a real disease, not just a make-believe one?

She explained that lupus is a chronic inflammatory disease of the connective tissues that hold the body together. I wasn't listening. "Lupus can affect the joints, tissue and other organs of the body," she continued. "I think you should go into the hospital for further testing before we discuss where to go from here. Also, it's important that you get some rest, and people don't rest as well at home as in the hospital."

My first reaction to her words was a giddy sensation of overwhelming relief. There was really a physical reason for the inconstant pain and all the illnesses, and they'd finally found it! It was *not* all in my head; all the doctors who had said that were wrong. I didn't even think about how serious this disease must be, to have caused all my symptoms, or that now there would be another hospital stay and still more tests. I just felt such a tremendous load off my mind that this doctor had discovered what was wrong with me, I thought my problems were as good as over. I had no idea of the long, tedious and devastating road ahead.

I agreed with the doctor about the "rest." I was exhausted, but I told her I would rest at home. I wanted no part of another hospital and I'd had enough tests. It had been two nights since I'd slept, and I just wanted to get out of the office. I was given a prescription for inflammation and one that would help my insomnia. I reluctantly agreed to use the medication for a trial period.

Later that day I met my girlfriend, Connie, for lunch. We had been close friends since my return to California, the kind of closeness that allowed us to share problems with each other.

I still didn't understand what lupus was, but by now I was starting to become a little worried. The word sounded so depressing. It was difficult to control the emotions that filled my mind.

"My blood tests showed lupus, whatever that is," I blurted. "The doctor wants me to have more tests."

Dear, sweet Connie listened with tear-filled eyes, and when I finished the story of my doctor visit, she put her hand over mine and squeezed it gently. Why was everyone acting so strangely about this disease? I found the doctor's and now Connie's reaction a little unnerving. I felt the first glimmer of fear.

"My sister has lupus," she said. "I've thought that might be what was wrong with you. I didn't want to be an alarmist, but that's why I kept urging you to see another doctor."

I stared at her in disbelief. "Your sister!" I gasped. "Now I remember. You did suggest a rheumatologist, but I had closed my mind to another doctor, and then I forgot what you had said . . . when I got ill again." I was stammering.

"Hey, that's okay," she assured me. "At least you got there. Now you'll get some help, and that's the important thing."

Connie went on to tell me more about lupus and of her sister's experience with the disease. I wondered what kind of malady this was that could so mysteriously and painfully restrict a person's life.

4
Changes in Lifestyle

It had been comforting to talk to Connie, someone who understood this disease that I had never heard of. However, it distressed me to be so uninformed about an illness that affected me. I wanted to learn as much as I could about lupus, and quickly.

At home that night I looked it up in the dictionary.

". . . a disease affecting the skin . . . scaly red patches, nodules which often ulcerate and leave scars." I didn't have any of those. Oh, no! Was that in my future? In a flurry, I opened a medical dictionary. I don't understand any of this . . . too technical . . . doesn't make any sense. My head was moving at a rapid speed, too fast to absorb what I read. Ah, here it is!

There are two forms of the disease. Discoid, the less serious type that affects the skin, was obviously not what I had. The other form, "systemic lupus erythematosus," was my problem. What a name! But that was it; I had the systemic type. At least I wouldn't be plagued by ugly skin eruptions.

Then I read some pamphlets from the doctor's office. I also searched through my books and found The Ann Landers Encyclopedia. Was it possible? Yes, there it was, in the section discussing arthritis. For years doctors had been telling me that I had arthritis, yet this was thc first reading I'd done on that disease.

My early childhood conditioning had told my head that the arthritis was a figment of my imagination, too. Also, until then, I had never realized how serious arthritis could be. I thought it was a disease of old age, of minor aches and pains. I was appalled to read, "Arthritis is the single largest crippler in the country. It is over one hundred diseases which involve inflammation or destruction of the joint." The article described the inflammation and joint pain that I had experienced over the years. My habit of pushing myself in order to forget my problems had only made my condition worse. Since I'd never taken the time to read about arthritis, it was small wonder I had never heard of lupus. I hadn't even considered arthritis enough of a danger to become better informed about it, despite the fact that I'd been told over and over that it was a problem for me. Perhaps if I'd been more knowledgeable, I would have gone to a rheumatologist sooner and saved myself years of pain.

I read further. "Among the diseases related to arthritis are even real killers—systemic lupus erythematosus, for example, at one time had a mortality rate of 30–50 percent within five years. . ." I was astounded. Fear now totally replaced the relief I had felt at finding out that my illness was not all in my mind. There was a sinking feeling in my stomach, and I had to force myself to continue reading. "A real killer," kept going through my mind. I ordered more pamphlets from the Arthritis Foundation.

For about ten days I was numb, in a state of shock. Then the material I had sent for arrived. I gathered up everything I had on lupus and sat down at the table, afraid of learning more, but realizing that I had to know the truth.

I read that this disease, commonly called lupus, was an "incurable, sometimes fatal disease" with remissions and flares that were typical of my medical past. Yes, I had been up and down like a yoyo. I would be well for months at a time, then deathly ill, then up again. My body was manic-depressive! Again I felt relief that my illness was not psychosomatic.

My entire medical history unfolded as I read—it was as if I were reliving all my years of illness. There it was, in black and white, described in detail. The vague symptoms that I had tried to explain to doctors; the weight loss, low-grade fever, dizziness, stiff neck, heaviness and swelling cause by inflammation, the joint pain, the weakness, the fatigue, aches throughout the body, and the pain that migrated from one area to another.

It explained that too much exposure to the sun could bring on a serious attack. No wonder I was so ill after a day at the beach in Honolulu. I looked well, and so did most lupus patients. It was all there; the confusing and debilitating pattern of lupus was the same pattern that had perplexed me and the doctors who had treated me. I learned that being sent from doctor to doctor was not unusual for victims of this disease.

But should it have confused the doctors, as well as me, a lay person? Wasn't it their business to detect syndromes and patterns of illnesses? Each of the almost countless specialists had treated only a part of me. Just one physician had finally recognized the signs of lupus.

I couldn't digest the rest of the information, but the treatment hit me like a dagger. "There is no known cure, but the disease can be controlled in most cases." Most cases! Controlled! I continued to read aloud. "Because lupus affects each patient differently, treatment varies considerably. Basically it involves rest, medication to ease pain, and drugs to reduce inflammation." The words medication and drugs glared up at me. I couldn't go through that again!

Then the word "incurable" hit me. No cure! My mind kept repeating this over and over. All the pain and weakness that I had hoped would disappear was going to be with me for the rest of my life. I wondered how long that would be. The thought was overpowering. I was terrified, and next I was overcome with an unbelievable fury.

One sleepless night after another, my anger was directed at the many doctors who had dismissed my complaints as psychosomatic while I suffered. I screamed in rage at the unnecessary anguish and depression I had gone through because the disease had not been detected. I pounded my pillow and cursed the doctors hysterically, remembering the drugs I had taken, the withdrawals I'd experienced. How could I have allowed all that to happen? Was it my fault? I didn't know. I wondered how many undiagnosed lupus victims never left a mental hospital.

I looked back on my Island days in disbelief. So much of my life had been at the mercy of others: their diagnoses, their opinions, their statements, which, once uttered, had taken control of my life. And now all their words were coming back to haunt *me*, not them. Why did I have to suffer for their mistakes? I lay on the bed and sobbed without restraint. The infections, fatigue, weakness and pain that traveled throughout my body, that I'd had so much trouble describing to doctors and to myself, were symptoms of lupus. They were not the imaginings of an emotionally disturbed person, as doctors had led me to believe. I had systemic lupus erythematosus. Lupus! Ugh!

"There's nothing wrong with you!" How many times had I heard that? And how many times had I left a doctor's office thinking they were right, that I was losing my mind. Then there were the doctors who had indiscriminately kept me on unnecessary medications, not knowing what else to do. They had taken the easy way out, and I had allowed all this to go on. No one had held a gun to my head, no one had forced me to take pills, no one had held my mouth open and poured the junk in. My thoughts raged on. I hated myself more than I hated the doctors. When would this fury go away? God, but it hurt.

Then one day Connie called. She had just heard a lupus patient being interviewed on national TV. "They flashed a hotline number to call," she related. "Why don't you write it down in case you want to talk to someone. It might help."

"Thanks a lot. I'll do that—tomorrow, I'll call," I lied.

"Also, my sister said to give you her number," Connie added. "I'm sure this is tough to accept and hard to live with. She'd like to help, maybe she can."

I wrote both numbers down, but I had no intention of calling anyone. I'd handle this myself.

What I remember about the next few weeks were the words "incurable" and "fatal" shattering my mind, and the feelings of fear, anger and denial that dominated my life. I ricocheted back and forth from one reaction to another, not able to accept that I could have something as serious as lupus and afraid that I did. The anger at myself was the worst, and I questioned why, over the past years, others couldn't have understood. And why didn't they understand what I was going through now. It never occurred to me that they couldn't understand because I hadn't told them. I still didn't know how to share my feelings with anyone. My mind, once again, kept floating in and out of reality. This just couldn't be happening to me.

For years I had deluded myself that my problems were all due to drugs, with a little arthritis thrown in. It was the arthritis I'd wanted controlled. "What are you talking about?" I reprimanded myself aloud. "Remember all the other problems? The constant fatigue that immobilized you for days, weeks—or was it months?

"True," I answered myself. True, also, that in the back of my mind was the belief that there was some other physical reason for my illnesses. Still, the sicker I got, the more I had held onto the conviction that everything was drug related, that once I was off drugs, I would eventually be all right. I had had hope. When I found out about lupus, I lost that hope. Until then, I had been struggling to stay sane, to wait it out, to get the drugs out of my system. But now that I realized my condition might be endless, I fell apart. My thinking was making me crazy! In addition, my faith went out the window and I was paralyzed by fear that overshadowed everything, even the physical pain.

The only way that I knew how to deal with this fear was to deny that there was anything wrong with me. I believed what I wanted to believe. I had to believe it. I still didn't want to face the fact that I had lupus. Things like that happened to other people, not to me. But I remembered saying that about drug addiction too, and I'd gone off drugs. My life had changed, and my emotional state had improved, but I was still sick. How could that be? It wasn't all emotional—that's how!

Yet, to change my thinking around at this point seemed impossible. I had been told that it was all in my head, and despite my unwillingness to accept that conclusion, I had learned to cope with it. I had believed that with time and patience, this would resolve itself. My "training" in the drug rehabilitation programs I'd been through had taught me that all I had to do was work hard at straightening out my life and stay away from drugs, never taking that first pill, and sooner or later, the nightmare would be over. But now I knew that wasn't true. Yes, I could deal with an emotional illness, if I saw an end in sight. But with lupus, there was no end but death. I had a truly serious illness. Oh God, I'd rather be losing my mind; please put the sickness back in my head. Please. PLEASE.

So I denied all of it, and pushed myself beyond any sane limitations. I thought that I could manage this illness by myself, but in truth I wasn't managing anything by myself. I had been told the importance of rest, and my body screamed for me to slow down. Instead I increased my activities and the pain escalated. I looked well, yet I did not know from day to day whether I would be able to stand up, let alone function with others. There were a few people that I confided in, that I told about the diagnosis. With the exception of Connie, no one had ever heard of the disease. I couldn't explain to them something that I really didn't understand myself. So, surrounded by my loving family and friends, I still felt alone with an illness I couldn't figure out, and one I was convinced I did not want to live with. I don't think I'll ever forget that time or the growing sense of panic and helplessness.

One day I got on my knees and prayed to a God that I'd almost forgotten. That night something compelled me to call the Lupus Hotline number. This was the turning point in my accepting and coping with the disease.

My hand shook as I dialed the number. My brain was numb, and I had no idea what I would say. A man answered, and I stuttered and stammered in an effort to explain why I was calling.

"Take your time," he said. "My name is Steve, and I've had lupus for over twenty years. I understand. It's going to be all right."

His voice was gentle and reassuring. For some reason, I believed him. A calmness came over me, and for the first time in weeks I began to relax. We talked about many things, but his words "I understand" were the most beautiful words I had ever heard. One person understood, really understood, how I felt without my saying anything. One person. That was all I needed then.

Steve recommended that I follow the doctor's suggestion to be hospitalized for observation and further tests. Later he gave me the phone number of a local chapter of a lupus organization in my area. Steve helped me learn to live with the emotional and physical aspects of this disease that had turned my life into a 24-hour nightmare.

"Oh God," I prayed. "Thanks for putting this wonderful loving man in my life. I'm so grateful. His pain is greater than mine, yet he held out his hand to me. Thanks—for everything." For the next two years Steve was to give me his much-needed caring support.

It was January 1980 when I entered the hospital. Since I was not in a drug or alcohol fog, this hospitalization was different, and I was aware of all that was happening. I felt more relaxed about being there, but I was also more tired than ever—inconceivable, but true, I reluctantly admitted to myself. But more important, this time there was a name for my problem; the reason for my being there was clear. My treatment had positive direction, and the treatment helped. My experience with drugs had left me with a determination to do without medication whenever possible, not to use it as a first resort. My new doctors respected this desire, and at that time, their prescribed treatment was bed rest, physical therapy and avoidance of stress.

"Stress is one of the primary causes of lupus flares," one doctor emphasized. "However, it's never too late to learn techniques for stress reduction, no matter how many years you've had stress in your life."

The doctors and I would work together. I would use

prayer and meditation instead of medications, and they would follow my progress closely. For me, this was the beginning of a spiritual approach to my illness. When the pain was intense, I felt God's arms holding and comforting me. The pain would ease, and in its place there was an emotional serenity that I had never felt before. No medication had ever done this.

Gradually my strength returned. I was able to eat properly, and the pain throughout my body diminished. When I returned home, I again had hope for the future. I no longer misused drugs and alcohol to treat myself. I honestly examined my motives before taking even an aspirin. Occasionally I became discouraged because there was still no answer for the severe pain that returned from time to time—no cure for this puzzling disease. I prayed that my condition would never reach the point where I would have to use drugs again.

Even though I openly acknowledged that I had lupus, part of me still clung to the rationalization that it was a mistake. This is just a temporary set-back, I fantasized. I'm not really sick.

My life began to change. In the summer of 1980 I started a new career as a writer.

I had begun writing lyrics and short stories at age seven, and continued as a teenager, also becoming absorbed in reading books of all kinds and dreaming of becoming a professional writer. But as an adult I had never had the courage, patience or time to launch this venture. I had needed a more consistent means of earning a living, so I had put my fantasy aside, out of my life as well as out of my mind. But now I had my chance.

I couldn't make a job committment, but my doctor had agreed that I could write at home as long as I paced myself. So I set out to do just that. I spent a lot of time alone, just me and my typewriter, my typewriter and me. Something good has come out of this illness, I beamed to myself. That old saying was true: when God closes one door, He opens another.

I listened to my body and geared my activities to my illness. Each morning when I awakened, I got on my knees before depressing thoughts could get to me.

"Dear God," I prayed, "just for today, I turn my life and my will over to Thee, praying only for knowledge of Your will for me and the power and humility to carry it out."

This simple prayer had been given to me by a friend. It worked for her and it was working for me. I felt a calmness and an inner energy that got me through many a trying day. Knowing I was following His will gave me the strength I needed to enjoy the day. It was like using an electric light switch. When the room was in darkness, I flipped a switch, the lights came on, and I had the power to see. I didn't question this power, but my dependency on it helped me to be more independent. So it was with turning my will over to God. Flipping the switch over to Him gave me the necessary strength to do what was in front of me and to know that, no matter what, everything would be all right. My reliance on His power made me feel more comfortable and secure, just as when I used a light switch.

Also, I had heard that meditation that helped healthy people could be especially beneficial to those with chronic illness and pain. But how does one meditate? My restless body wouldn't be still, and my head wouldn't shut up—I couldn't sit quietly for even one minute. I tried everything. I read about meditation, then I asked everyone I knew who used it as a means to serenity, "How do you meditate?" And in the end I did it in a way that worked for me. When my mind was especially active, watching the flickering flame of a candle helped, but it was a slow process. Quieting my mind wasn't easy. It kept wandering off to what I needed to do that day, and it made me nervous to sit silently. In the beginning I could only do it for two minutes at a time, but gradually, I worked up to ten minutes by reading spiritual passages each morning. I put my answering machine on so as not to be disturbed, and if my thoughts wandered, I persistently brought them back. I was determined not to allow anything to interfere with this morning meditation. It was hard work, and my impatience plagued me. "What's ten minutes a day out of your life?" I kept asking myself. "You can certainly give ten minutes a day towards feeling better." I was willing to try.

A friend gave me a subscription to the *Daily Word*. It was there that I found a prayer on healing that worked especially well to calm my body. I used it every day:

> Dear God, here is my body. Fill it with Your healing life. Here is my mind. Immerse it in Your true peace. I am one with You and You are one with me. I cannot be separated from Your radiant life which is even now vitalizing and renewing me, making me every whit whole.
>
> I let go yesterday's concepts and accept the concept of wholeness. I let go yesterday's binding thoughts of weakness, age, imperfection of any kind. I feel alive, I look alive, I am alive. I enjoy perfect health now.
>
> I know that even as I am one with Your healing presence, so are my dear ones and all people one with Your life, one with Your healing power. I see those for whom I pray as truly alive. I see each one filled with your radiant life, vitalized, renewed, at peace in mind and body.

As the months went by, I learned new techniques and was able to increase my meditation time to half an hour. Allowing my thoughts to drift back to Honolulu, I put my mind in a quiet place, a warm place with lovely blue skies and an ocean breeze. Honolulu, where my life had become a nightmare, now remained as a place in my mind where I could relax and prepare for the day.

After prayer and meditation, it was on to the shower. There, like the magic of meditation, the water washed away the pain that had settled in my muscles during the night. I felt as if a massive weight had been lifted from my body, a dense veil taken from my eyes. My head cleared—the throbbing in my temples was no longer there. Oh, how I remembered that endless pounding in my head and throughout my body. It was gone. I could feel God's arms around me, holding me, dissolving all my fears and helping me carry my painful load.

Each night I thanked God for the day and prayed for the health and happiness of my family and friends. And then I slept without pills. This miracle never ceased to amaze me, and I woke up happy to be alive and eager for the new day. My life improved. This spiritual program was working for me. With meditation and prayer I had been given something more important than physical well-being—I had peace-of-mind. My faith saw me through the bad days, and there is nothing like chronic pain to make one grateful for the good days. I resolved that, with God's help, I would one day get this disease under control. But the road curved, it got bumpy and lengthy, and I faltered along the way.

At times I refused to admit there was anything wrong with me, pushing myself and then suffering the consequences. I could not completely accept the fact that I had some mysterious, incurable disease that with alarming speed could, and frequently did, immobilize me with pain and fatigue. Whenever a job had to be done, my lifetime habit had been to finish that job, no matter how tired I became. That had to change—I had to rest *before* I got tired. That would be some neat trick!

"Put some relaxation in your life," my doctor advised. "Rest and relaxation! Try it!"

"R and R" was something we joked about; I hadn't realized how difficult those things were to do. They sounded simple, and they *were* simple. But they weren't *easy*.

"It's never easy to change lifetime habits," a friend reminded me.

How true, I thought, especially for someone like me who had never allowed time for resting, and now felt guilty when I did.

The next thing to change were my eating habits. While there were no specific dietary recommendations for the management of lupus, my doctor had suggested eliminating certain foods, such as sugar, salt, wheat, caffeine, and tomatoes. He also stressed that a well-balanced diet was essential, and that meant a diet consisting of moderate quantities of all other types of food. I was to avoid fad diets since they were unbalanced and nutritionally inadequate, being more detrimental than beneficial.

If nutrition played such an important role in well-being, than I would learn to eat properly, I decided, after doing more reading on the subject of good health. My younger daughter, Annie, a healthy vegetarian and knowledgeable in nutrition and diet, became my helper.

"Mom, what you eat has a direct influence on how you feel," she said. "If you're not providing the right kinds of nutrients, or if you're providing waste materials to your body instead of nutrients, your body will not be as energetic because it's working extra hard without the right fuel."

"Waste materials?" I asked. "You mean empty calories, like sugar, that provide fast, short-term energy, but no real nourishment?"

"Right. Maybe you could make a list of the best foods to eat to get your carbohydrates, fats, proteins and minerals. Oh yes, and vitamins, of course, but a balanced diet will have all the vitamins you need."

"Good idea! I know a little about all that, but I need to learn more. And I'll put the list on my refrigerator door!"

I made my list, keeping in mind that a balanced diet consists of about sixty-five percent carbohydrates—mainly the complex carbohydrates like green vegetables, potatoes and cereals, not sugars such as candy and sweets—then twenty percent fat and ten to fifteen percent proteins.

"Throw away all those fast food cakes," my daughter had emphasized. "Sugar, like you said, provides fast energy since it's absorbed rapidly, but complex carbohydrates provide a more constant supply. They metabolize more slowly. You need carbohydrates for energy; they're converted into glucose, which means energy, energy for breathing, moving, thinking, keeping the body warm."

"Sounds good to me!" I agreed.

Annie took it further, one step at a time, and soon I had eliminated salt, my all-time favorite. It took weeks of bemoaning the tastelessness of things before I began to enjoy the natural flavor of foods. By then I had replaced my destructive eating habits with a well-balanced diet consisting mainly of fresh vegetables, cereals, fish, poultry, some potatoes and whole wheat bread, non-fat milk and non-fat cheese. Ounce for ounce, cheese has twice the protein of meat!

"It also contains calcium and phosphorous and

other important vitamins," Annie reminded me. "But be careful not to overdo on cheeses—cholesterol, you know—and use the non-fat or low-fat kind."

From health books, I learned that improper diet is believed to be one of the principal causes of cardiovascular disease, the leading cause of death in the United States. I continued reading; "the circulation of the blood to the organs of the body is vital to life." The arteries must not become clogged. Calcium deposits over a period of years cause hardening of the arteries and are a factor in the aging process. Well, some of this is to be expected as one grows older, I mused, but cholesterol deposits in the arteries, called plaque, are usually controllable by diet and exercise. So, I began to watch my diet, avoiding foods high in salt, sugar, cholesterol and fat. Easy to say, but not as easy to do.

"Also, don't forget the importance of water," Annie suggested one day. "No food is as important to the body."

"I didn't know water was considered a food."

"Sure. It's taken into the body as a part of other food elements, as well as in drinking. A loss of only ten percent of the body's water can cause death. But the good news is that there is water in all food, even dry bread. Anyway you ought to drink a little more than your thirst requires. I know you don't drink alcohol anymore. What about coffee?"

"That's next, I guess," I answered. "I heard that caffeine causes all sorts of problems, like irregular heartbeat, insomnia, high blood pressure, stomach problems, and possible cancer of the pancreas. Also, it was one of the things a doctor once suggested that lupus patients eliminate from their diet. It's worth a try."

That day I changed to decaffeinated coffee and herbal teas.

"I have this giant headache," I complained to my girlfriend, Susan. "It feels like the top of my head is exploding, coming off!"

"That's caffeine withdrawal," she said. "Same thing happened to me when I stopped coffee. You have to withdraw slowly."

My doctor verified what she said, and my headache disappeared when I put caffeine back into my body. I started again with non-caffeinated drinks, only this time I did it gradually, not making a sudden changeover.

Smoking was the next to go. That was without a doubt the hardest change I ever made. I knew all the facts, but reading all those statistics upset me so much I smoked even more. I was addicted to cigarettes, and logic had nothing to do with anything! People tried to get me to stop smoking by reminding me of facts such as, "cigarettes kill nearly 500,000 Americans each year, which means that one in four deaths is caused by cigarette smoking." My children, in their early teens, tried every means to convince me. I smoked more. One time my son came up with the idea of barricading the smoke in my room by putting towels around the bedroom door, then filling the room with burning incense. I coughed my way out of that one.

"Please stop smoking," thirteen-year-old Annie had pleaded dramatically. "You're killing yourself! And what about me? You'll die and I'll be all alone!" She had cried hysterically and run from the smoke-filled room.

The truth in her emotional outburst did not penetrate my consciousness. Also, I didn't stop to think what I was doing to the lungs of the three most important people in my life, my children. Anger and guilt raged inside me at their insinuations, and I continued to smoke more and more, all day long, even in the shower. Even though I had reached the point where smoking no longer satisfied or relaxed me, I just couldn't stop. I read books, tried self-help programs and stop-smoking programs, tried everything. My children tried everything. Nothing worked.

I listened to tapes, kept records, and one time had stopped for several weeks. Another time I had cut down to one cigarette a day, but after several weeks, that one cigarette had led to one pack, and soon I was smoking four packs a day, which was even more than when I'd begun the plan. One day, a friend told me about a five-day program that had worked for her. Okay, Leading Cause of Preventable Death, okay, Cigarette Smoking, this is it. This is going to work! At least it couldn't hurt.

For some reason, the Seventh Day Adventist's simple program worked for me. But it was not easy. It took weeks of painful withdrawals and months before I could do anything without thinking about a cigarette. I threw away all my stray cigarettes and allowed no smoking in my apartment, and no matter how nervous I became or how much I craved a cigarette, no matter what, I just didn't take one. I meditated several times a day. Gradually the craving diminished and I knew the worst was over. I had become a non-smoker.

"I'm sure glad you stopped smoking," my daughter said. "Nicotine, like alcohol, causes the platelets in the blood to stick together, interfering with capillary circulation. This makes arthritic pain worse, and you have enough problems without giving yourself more pain."

"Amen to that!" I laughed. "And let's not forget the other dangers of smoking."

"I know them all," Annie giggled. "I've been trying to get you to quit so long. There's heart and artery disease, lung cancer, increased risks of blood clots and osteoporosis..."

"Enough!" I interrupted with a laugh. "Seems I've

heard all that before! *I'm* happy that I stopped smoking, too, but believe me, it was the hardest thing I've ever done."

"I know, and I'm proud of you."

"Thanks. Well, gotta go now and get some rest."

"Good idea. I'll talk to you later."

"Right. Goodnight."

Slowly the good things I put into my body and the harmful things I eliminated had a positive effect. My health improved, my thinking improved, and I felt better. If I could just keep my mind functioning even on the days when my body didn't, I would be all right. I just knew that.

Thus, faced with a disabling disease, I had become willing to change the negative aspects of my life, to do whatever was necessary to live a quality life, lupus or not. I made adjustments and changed my thinking regarding stressful situations. While others lived with everyday stress, the toll it could exact on me would be hospitalizations or death. I had to simplify my life.

So I began to adjust to my new life and its limitations. One of the hardest parts was not being able to make any commitments. I'd always had difficulty saying "no." I felt guilty when I refused a simple dinner invitation because it was too painful to get dressed. Now there were many times I would have to break appointments with my family and friends, or not make any plans at all, because I never knew from day to day how I would feel. I could wake up in the morning feeling fine and by afternoon not be able to move out of bed, with an indescribable bone-tiredness. There was never a 24-hour period in which I was totally free of pain.

I thought I had accepted these facts and restrictions, and prepared to get on with my life. After all, I had this disease called lupus. "Pace yourself, Beverly,"

I screamed to empty walls. "Pace yourself!" I could feel the anger and irritability building up again.

"I have so much trouble explaining to others why I can't do things I used to do, or run around in the same way," I commented to Susan. "I'm so tired of having to do that. Why can't I say 'no' without long explanations or excuses? I guess I'm afraid of what people will think."

"I understand," she responded, "and I'll bet your family and other friends do, too. We accept it. Maybe it's you who is not accepting."

Nonsense! I thought, but I knew she believed it was true. Still I wondered how friends and family really felt. Did they think I was just making excuses?

This concern kept me in a constant state of anxiety, and it wasn't until years later that I realized Susan was right. It was I, not others, who remained intolerant of the constraints my disease put on me.

Still, I was happy. Little things gave me great joy, and I kept writing. In 1980, I sold my first story. It reminded me of giving birth to a child, including the pain before birth and the pure delight afterwards. I went around smiling all day, even in the shower, giddy with excitement and deluged with gratitude. Thank you, God. Thank you, God, I murmured. My life was full; everything was finally falling into place. I can deal with the pain and weakness, I repeated over and over again. It meant pacing myself, eating properly, exercising regularly, changing my life style, and taking care to avoid the sun. But I could do it—I would! Serenely confident, I believed that I would never require further hospitalization if I followed my new life-rules. My tranquility would have been shattered if I'd had a crystal ball!

I had chosen a highly competitive and lonely profession, one that kept my mailbox filled with rejection letters, and my mind kept slipping into a pitfall of depression. Then in January of 1981 Parks Herzog was put into my life. The confidence that he expressed in my writing ability spurred me on to continue with my work. He gave me the encouragement I needed, and he became the friend who would always be there for me. Maybe, just maybe, I would be able to write the story of what had happened to me since I had become ill.

With this new reason for living, I started to work on that story. And things went rather well for me—until that summer.

5
A Setback

It was June 1981. The city had one of the worst heat waves in years. It lasted for weeks, with temperatures soaring to 105 degrees. The entire city suffered; hospitals filled to capacity and patients overflowed into the halls. There was no relief, even at night. The lucky ones worked and lived in air-conditioned places, but I was not one of those lucky ones. I lived close to the ocean, where air-conditioning seemed unnecessary—until this summer.

For five days I sweltered with just a small fan. I tried a larger fan, but it succeeded only in shattering my nerves with its noise and the circulation of hot air. The heat oppressed me, making sleep nearly impossible, and I could barely breathe. Then on the afternoon of the fifth day, it began. I felt paralyzed with fatigue; my eyes wouldn't focus and everything blurred. I couldn't see the numbers on the telephone dial. Where are my glasses? I need my glasses to find my glasses! I panicked. Ah, here they are! The room continued to spin.

I stumbled through the day as frantic fear built up inside me. Somehow time passed, each minute an eternity, but I didn't call anyone. I couldn't share my defeat. Old recordings plagued my mind, and gritting my teeth, I forgot about prayer and meditation. I could handle it myself.

That evening I sat in my living room chair, rocking

back and forth, wondering when this, too, would pass, as the saying goes. My eyes still wouldn't focus, and they hurt from straining to see all day. I couldn't remember when I had slept; I was too exhausted to eat and too uneasy to relax.

On the sixth day, a strange and frightening pain appeared, like a heavy weight pressing on my chest, suffocating me. I ached all over, and when I stood up, my legs were rubbery. But lying down, my body vibrated with pain. My heart was beating irregularly and I could hardly catch my breath.

"You're having a lupus flare, probably aggravated by the heat," Dr. Reed said in the examining room. "Also, we'd best have a cardiologist check you."

Impossible as it seemed, the weakness and pain felt more severe than in the past, and my breathing problems frightened me. My sedimentation rate was up, my blood pressure a mere 80/58, and I had a low-grade fever. A cardiac ultrasound was performed because of my chest pain, and the findings showed a mitral valve prolapse—something else I had never heard of.

The doctor informed me that the symptoms may include heart palpitations, shortness of breath and stabbing pains that may last hours or even days.

"That's exactly what I've been having," I acknowledged. "But this stabbing pain moves around so often, each day a different place! So I didn't mention it to you. I also felt as if I were suffocating. If I didn't ignore some of these things, I'd be calling you daily with some kind of complaint."

"Actually, this is a very common condition. Studies show that at least six percent of all women have it."

I learned that in mitral valve prolapse one or both of the mitral valve flaps are enlarged and some of their supporting strings are too long. What this meant was that when the heart contracts, the mitral valve flaps do not close smoothly or evenly. Instead, part of one or both flaps collapse backward into the left atrium, sometimes allowing a small amount of blood to leak backward through the valve.

During this hospitalization, I had complete gastrointestinal testing, better known as the G.I. series. And even better known to patients as those nauseating barium tests—ugh!—and various other things. The results uncovered a hiatus hernia in my esophagus, which accounted for much of my discomfort, especially the feelings of suffocation.

Also, at this time, one of the doctors reiterated what I had read when I first heard of lupus. He explained that lupus causes inflammation of the connective tissue. "The connective tissue supports the cells of the body," he said, "somewhat like mortar connects and supports bricks of a house. When the membranes and connective tissue around the heart become inflamed, it causes a condition known as pericarditis, which is inflammation of the lining of the heart. Pain then results from friction created with movement.

"Pleurisy is also quite common in lupus patients. This is an irritation of the membranes lining the chest, causing painful breathing. Related symptoms are shortness of breath or rapid heartbeat. There may be an accumulation of fluid in the chest cavity from the inflammatory changes. In addition to the organ linings, the disease can directly damage the organs themselves. It's important that the inflammation be reduced.". I started the necessary drug therapy to alleviate the inflammation in my body and to prevent further damage.

"Rest!" Dr. Reed again reminded me. "This is very important. Your body needs more of that now."

This created no problem in the hospital; exhaustion had set in and I slept most of the next three days.

Soon my appetite returned and the pain in my chest and throughout my body diminished. I began to feel human again.

But on the morning of the fifth day I suddenly had a relapse. Someone had left my chart in the room, and I jumped at the opportunity to read it. Lupus! Cold chills went through me. There was that word again. I dropped the chart and climbed back into bed. Again, I was hit with the realization that I was sick! Very sick. I can't live with that, I sobbed. I could hardly believe the illness, yet alone live with it. This happened to other people, not to me.

My anger exhausted me and I became weak with despair. Call someone, tell someone how you feel, anyone! this prudent voice inside me said. But one of my old ideas came back with sudden force: no matter how you feel, be cheerful. Nobody loves a complainer. You shouldn't tell anyone you hurt; it's not nice. What will people think? They won't like you. Lie! People must think you're in control of everything. You must be perfect—don't show any weakness. This recording played over and over in my mind, and I decided not to share my feelings with anyone.

I remained in the hospital twenty-six days. When anyone visited me, I suppressed the tears that threatened to expose my feelings. My family and friends loved me through those weeks, but I felt as if God had abandoned me. That painful empty feeling had returned. Isolated and alone, even in the midst of people who cared about me, I couldn't confide in anyone, not even Steve. After two years I should be on top of the situation. Hadn't I tried so hard? Wasn't I supposed to be able to handle anything? Wasn't I supposed to be perfect? Irrational attitudes from years ago flooded my mind, and I stopped praying and took matters back into my own hands. I forgot about the light switch.

I couldn't let anyone see any weakness in me. I thought that I was letting everyone down by feeling frightened and alone, and so I became even more afraid and more lonely. Where was that fight? All gone, I moaned to myself; I'm just too tired. Depression and self-pity filled my mind. I had given up; I couldn't accept this illness. I'm so tired, I exclaimed.

That night I lay curled up on the hospital bed, twisting back and forth. I thought about praying for the pain in my body and my mind to go away, but I didn't. So the fear stayed with me, creeping through my being even as I slept, invading my dreams, turning them into nightmares. All I saw was the doctor's notation on the chart, the reason for my admittance to the hospital. Lupus! My emotions and fatigue overshadowed everything else, even the physical pain. Too weary to do anything else, I let go and again became willing to turn my life, with all its problems, over to the care of God. I got on my knees, not an easy task in the hospital, and I prayed. "Thy will, not mine," I screamed inwardly, then out loud murmured it quietly. "Help me. Please help me." The tears finally came.

I climbed back into bed and lay there with my eyes shut, letting the peace take over my shattered emotions. Then from out of nowhere, it occurred to me that Steve had given me the number to call for a local lupus support group. What had I done with it? Wait a minute, don't panic, I reminded myself. I searched my wallet and emptied the contents of my purse on the bed, looking for it. Why couldn't I ever find phone numbers? There it was! Should I call? "Beverly, just do it!" I yelled out loud to an empty room. Reluctantly, I picked up the phone and made my first contact with a member of a lupus self-help group. Another door had opened for me, though I didn't realize it at the time.

"We have a meeting next week," the woman from the rap group said. "Would you like someone to pick you up?"

"Well, I don't know," I said, reluctant to make any commitment. "I think I'll be going to stay with some friends out of town when I leave the hospital. Maybe in a couple of months, though."

One week seemed too soon after being in bed for three weeks, I rationalized. Actually it was a subliminal fear that motivated me to dream up the phone excuse, and later I realized I was afraid of being with other sick people. Also, in my state of mind, I didn't think anything could possibly do any good. How could a rap group help? By the time I got home, I had decided not to go.

One day shortly after leaving the hospital, I was having lunch with Susan. "Let's go shopping," she suggested. "I know you've been having a rough time. Maybe buying something new will help, and anyway, it'll be fun."

Well, lunch had been fun, but from then on, it was strictly downhill. In the department store I sat in the dressing room, surrounded by clothes, and cried. I can't even go out for two hours without being overcome by weakness, I reflected. How can I continue with this daily fatigue, the pain . . .

"I'm exhausted!" I blurted out as Susan walked into the room. "Just once I'd like to go shopping and try on a dress without feeling as if I'm lifting a thousand pounds when I raise my arms."

With this outburst, I panicked. I wanted to go home. My clothes weighed a ton. Had to get home and get my clothes off. My mind raced in confusion.

"Bev, it's okay," Susan comforted. "It's been a long day and we did too much. Let's get out of here—just leave everything."

That night at home, pain ravaged my body and mind. Then came the utter depths; the emotional upheaval I had experienced when I first heard of lupus had started again. It hit me with such suddenness, I was totally unprepared for the depression that took hold of my mind. What was the point of living. Once more I felt alone with a disease that baffled me, but false pride kept me from calling the lady from the rap group. Then I thought of calling Parks, but I remembered that he was 3000 miles away on a business trip. I couldn't tell him of my despair. Actually, I didn't want to tell anyone—what would they think of me? God, I wished I had a pill, a whole bottle of pills! I had suffered enough. Maybe I could go into the kitchen and turn on the gas—that was supposed to be painless—then I wouldn't be a bother to anyone ever again.

The loud ringing of the telephone jarred me back to reality. Hesitantly, I answered it.

"Beverly," began the soft voice of a woman. "This is Laura. I spoke to you several weeks ago in the hospital, remember? About going to a lupus rap group?"

"Sure," I stammered. I was stunned. "How nice to hear from you."

"Thanks. How're you doing?"

"Fine," I said, and then I felt guilty. Be honest, an inner voice said. I tried. "To tell the truth, I'm *really* glad you called because actually I'm a little depressed."

"I'm sorry to hear that," she said. "Anything I can do to help?"

"I don't think so, but it's good to talk to you."

"You know, lupus is not an easy disease to live with. That's one of the things we talk about at our rap groups. Would you be interested in going?"

"Well..." I tried to think of some way to decline. Every week. A commitment. The fear came back.

"There's one this Saturday," Laura interjected. "I can have you picked up, if you like. Why not at least try it? You don't have to make a commitment for every week. Just see how you like it."

She's reading my mind. How did she know, I wondered.

"It's just that I'm not sure I have the strength for anything like that," I said. I would be with others who had lupus. I was afraid, but what was I afraid of? Things couldn't get any worse. My life was a shambles now, and I certainly didn't want to live like this. Willing to go to any lengths—where had I heard that? Was I that willing? My mind drifted back to Laura's voice.

"We're not doctors, but maybe we can help you deal with the many emotional aspects of this disease," she continued. Her voice was kind. "We all understand how you feel—we've been there. Think about it. Maybe you can get to at least one meeting."

"I'll try." I made no promises, but carefully put the address away.

Laura also gave me the phone number of someone who lived nearby. "She will be glad to take you. Just give her a call, and if that doesn't work out, call me back."

Laura and I had not met, but I knew she cared about me. My suicidal thoughts had vanished, my thinking turned around by one phone call. Thank you, God, I whispered. I vowed to remember the healing power of calling someone if I ever got that despondent again.

I recalled another remedy for depression, one that Susan had told me. "When you get depressed, write a grateful list," she had said.

"Why can't I just think about the things I'm grateful

for," I had asked. "Why write it? That's so much trouble."

"It's not the same," she said. "There's something magic about putting it on paper, and better yet reading it to someone. It works. Try it!"

So I did, again and again, when I remembered, and it always got me out of negative thinking, always changed how I felt inside. When I'm feeling grateful, it's impossible to be negative. But you forget that, dummy! It's not too much trouble, not for the benefits you get. Just take a pen and paper and do it now!

I wrote, "I'm grateful for: my hands, this pencil, the paper..." and so it went until I finally felt the change seep through me. "Grateful for my children, my family, my friends, my eyes, hands, legs, and my body—such as it is!" Ah, at last, a smile crept through. If I could just laugh at myself, I'd be all right. Don't take yourself or life so seriously, I reminded myself. I didn't want to go back to that time in Honolulu, back to the negativity I'd experienced for so long. I was lucky—I now knew what was wrong with me. I had a diagnosis, and like it or not, I would learn to accept it and get on with living.

It was September when I finally attended a rap group meeting, the first of many. I went filled with apprehension and my old fear of being around sick people, and these were strangers. Besides, I still could not say the word "lupus" without cringing.

The meeting took place in a private home and everyone was friendly. They looked so happy and healthy, I could hardly believe they were lupus patients. Then I remembered what people had said to me; "Bev, you look so well, you can't be sick."

I was introduced to the group and asked if I wanted to share. At first it distressed me to talk about myself in front of a group of people that I didn't know, but there was an undeniable feeling of warmth and love in that room. Suddenly the words came, almost without effort, as if someone else were talking. I felt free and devoid of fear as I told them about my experiences and feelings, then I listened intently as they shared theirs. They were talking about themselves, but they were telling my story of anguish and pain. That heavy weight again lifted from me—there were others who lived with this disease and who knew how I felt.

When the meeting ended that morning, we all exchanged phone numbers. As I left I smiled at one of the women and she returned the smile. I walked through the living room and stood quietly at the front door, then turned and looked at those who had gathered in little groups to talk with one another. I recognized that these people were my friends. I intuitively knew that on my bad days I could pick up the phone and call any one of them. Unbelievably, in two short hours they had become an important part of my life. I no longer felt alone.

One day Susan drove me to my parents' home. Weakness and light-headedness kept me from driving that ten miles.

"I love to drive," I confided, "but ten minutes behind the wheel and my body starts to hurt. Sometimes it's difficult to lift my foot to step on the brake. It's frightening and frustrating."

"Then don't drive," she responded matter of factly. "It's that simple."

"That's easy to say," I said with a laugh. "But it's really hard for me to do. I feel so guilty saying that I can't do something and I hate asking someone to drive me any place—you know that. I wouldn't be going today if you hadn't asked me. It's wearisome to keep making excuses, even if they aren't really excuses. Sometimes it makes me want to cry, and at other times I'm so frustrated and angry I want to scream at my body."

"Like you said, you aren't making excuses," she agreed. "Those are the facts that you have to accept. You've got to stop worrying about what other people think, stop being such a people-pleaser. It's either that, and damn the consequences, or suffer, and you're the one who suffers, no one else. And who cares, anyway? If people don't understand, that's their problem, not yours! Your problem is taking care of yourself. End of lecture!"

I laughed and Susan grinned back. "Honestly, Bev, I didn't mean to be so dogmatic," she said. "I just hate to see you being so hard on yourself. I care about you."

"I know," I said. "Thanks. That's all good advice, too. I have to start practicing it. And by the way, I appreciate your caring."

The following week I was reminded of the truth of her words, and I found out the hard way that I had more to learn about saying "no." Some of my other friends had invited me on a week-end trip. However, it had been one of those bad weeks for me and I decided to rest at home.

"Why don't you change your mind and join us," Joan urged. "Maybe a change of scenery will do you good."

"I don't think I can make the drive," I said, beginning to feel irritable. "I'm a little tired." Speak up, dummy! A little tired—you're exhausted, my head reprimanded.

"Oh, come on. We'll stop along the way and break the trip up, so you won't get tired. It'll be fun."

I succumbed. The people-pleaser in me won out, and true to Susan's words of wisdom, I paid the price. When I returned from that fun week-end, I came back to another hospitalization, and back to a favorite dream of mine, where I would confide in my doctor and tell him how I felt. In my thoughts the monologue went something like this:

"Doctor, I wonder if you're aware of just how difficult it is for me to get through the day, doing simple things, just taking care of myself? My vision is bad—so blurry that my head becomes disjointed and confused. It's painful to hold a toothbrush. Even my hair hurts. Dizzy and lightheaded, I go from task to task. This is an almost daily occurrence and it's getting worse. When it happens, my eyes close—no matter what I'm doing, I can't keep them open. Fatigue sets in, indescribable lupus fatigue. My muscles become weak, and my body slumps. Wherever I am, I must go to sleep, only then comes the blessed relief from the pain.

"And then to the other extreme," I would continue nonstop, "I get insomnia. That's also a part of this disease. You've told me that so many times, and it surely must be true, for I have difficulty sleeping when I'm in a flare, and the insomnia increases the intensity of the flare. It's a vicious circle.

"What I would like is just 24 hours free from the 'spacey' feeling and the pain. I would like to feel that my feet are on terra firma and not on stilts, with me looking for a place to put each stilt. I want to walk with ease, not fall over my feet and lose my balance as if I were drunk. Did I stop drinking just to walk like a drunk because of lupus? All I want from you, Doctor, is to help me get through the day, one day, this day. And to understand how I feel."

It was two years before I shared those feelings with a doctor. For now, I again told the doctors of my symptoms, but not of my difficulties in living with those symptoms. I was still keeping that a big secret—and that secret along with my unexpressed anger was killing me.

But then, I was good at keeping secrets. Throughout the years of hospitalizations in Honolulu, I never let my family know of my many illnesses, although my sister Cindy and I kept in close touch. She became my link to family activities, and she always knew where I was. She patiently followed my escapades in and out of hospitals. I trusted her to keep me informed and to keep my confidence, and she never let me down. I felt lucky to have such a close relationship with my sister, lucky and ever grateful. I knew many families where that kind of love didn't exist.

In 1980, after I was diagnosed with lupus, Cindy returned the letters I had written her from the hospital in Honolulu.

"If you could get through that bad time with drugs and withdrawals," she said, "you can get through anything. You'll make it! I know you will; just let me know what I can do to help. I love you."

"Thank you. I love you, too." I hid the letters under the mattress of my bed, without reading them. And there they remained until one day when I moved into a new apartment. The moving men called my attention to the letters, and I stuffed them in my purse to read later.

That night, in the quiet of my living room, I opened the first envelope, thinking of my sister's words as I read:

February 20, 1977

Dear Cindy,

Well, here I am—not knowing how I got to this point or why. Should keep a diary and send daily to you, so I don't forget. (Just what you need! A daily account of this place!) Actually, don't know how I'll ever forget, but I would hate to get into this Hell again.

Wow, would I ever hate to be here again! Once is too much.

Hard to concentrate—they started medication last night. I really felt "way-out."

It was good talking to you. Hope I didn't say anything "wrong"—can't remember because I was in such a fog then. These meds make me crazy. Whoops, better be careful of that word! Anyway, I didn't mean that anyone was putting pressure on me. I do that very nicely all by myself.

I hope Katherine is feeling better and that you were able to go on your trip. Have fun!

It's Saturday—has been for hours *and* for most of this letter. You would *not* believe the "nutty" conversations I've been having with the others here. Oh well, at least we're laughing a lot. Though really I wish I could cry. You know all those questions Annie's been asking and we decided are universal (like the whole world's falling apart, etc.) Well, I am loudly asking, too! Boy, I really am talking a lot. Trying to find *me*. Who am I? Where am I? Not really me—someone else had invaded my body! Damn! The body snatcher? Seems long ago, I was looking for me. How does that song go? What is wrong with me? I can't remember. What *is* wrong with me anyway? What a question!

Honey, I am dizzy (don't laugh!) and very tired. It's difficult to write anymore. Really only wanted to write a few words anyway, to let you know that I am doing okay and am getting good care in this place. Don't know if this letter will be reassuring or not!—but will mail it anyway because I may not write again for a while. It's *really* very difficult. My hand seems to go one way and my way-ahead thoughts another. Hence this scribble.

Thank you for everything—as I said, it *really* was good to talk to you, and very helpful.

Kiss the girls for me. I miss you all very much! My love to you and Fred and all my family.

Bev

P.S. I really do feel better every day.

I had to laugh at the postscript, remembering the fear each day brought and that I had felt far from better.

Cindy had given me three letters. The next one was from my girlfriend, Elly. It was dated February 19, 1977. I could still remember with horror how I had felt inside during those drug-filled days. It made me realize that I had indeed come a long way—I was no longer filled with that incredible fear and dazed confusion. I opened Elly's short letter to my sister and smiled as I pictured my dear friend.

Dear Cindy,

Although we don't know each other, I will let you know that I saw Beverly this afternoon and she is alright. She asked me to mail this to you. Thought you would like the pictures. I am staying in her apartment until she can come back from the hospital. Let's hope that will be soon. She gained four pounds in two days! Isn't that wonderful. Please give my regards to your parents.

Sincerely,
Elly Ras

The last letter I discovered had been written over a month later. My handwriting had become small and cramped. I had felt more uncertain than ever about my future.

Dear Cindy,

I left the hospital Friday, March 11, after 22 days. Three days later I moved into an alcohol and drug addiction facility. Been meaning to write you sooner—thought about it daily! It's nearly a 24-hour program here. Starting at 6 a.m., we work at something almost around the clock. Or at least it seems that way. Still leaves plenty of time to be lonely! But not much time for writing. There's also been my frame of mind and the uncertainty of what I would do kept me from writing. Many things still uncertain, but feel hopeful the program here will help me, if I really work at it. Don't know how long I'll be here—it may be six months or however long it takes. I'm going to discontinue the answering service as Elly has been and will continue to stay in my apartment—until—who knows? I'll let you know if that changes. Until then, she's there to take calls, when she's not at work, and picks my mail up at my post office box, too. She's such a lovely friend.

I'm starting a university correspondence class in psychology, via the radio. I'll be getting help here in working toward becoming a counselor or something in that field. There are approximately sixty people living here. We all share in the work—cleaning, cooking (!), yard, etc. Also many daily different classes and therapy groups. Will explain it all later—too much to write now. I've been very ill and am just beginning to feel a little better. I can only hope I'm doing the right thing by being here. It seemed my only choice at this point.

At first they turned me down for entry—didn't think I could take the pressure. My doctor agreed with them. However I did not. So I kept calling them while I was still in the hospital, and was given a second interview, and accepted. The program is in the process of undergoing many changes. Anyway, as I said, I'll try to write you more about what's going on as soon as possible. That might be months!—know you understand.

Mother sent me a newspaper clipping of Danielle eating spaghetti and it told of your hosting a Parent Education meeting at the school. I'm proud of you and of all you're doing. And Danielle looks so beautiful. Since I now have her picture, how about sending me ones of Katherine, Ilaina and Julia? Then I'll have your whole brood! I miss you all very much! Of course, I miss my children the most. Speaking of them, Annie phoned me when I was in the hospital (answering service took her call). I tried to phone her, but no answer. However, I received a letter from her that I think was written after the call so perhaps she just called to see how I was feeling. I think Mother told the children that I was not well since I received letters from Jeff and Adrienne also, saying that they hoped I was feeling better. To my knowledge, no one knows about the hospital. I answered their letters, but have not yet written *any* of my children about the hospital or my illness or of where I'm "at" now. I want to, but I'm uncertain as to what to write. I don't want to say anything that will hurt or worry them. I know they have their own lives and problems and I want them to feel and know that I'm available to help, whenever they want or need me. Also, I don't want them relating to my problems. Nor, in any way be a burden to them. On the other hand, I want to be honest with them and not "lie by omission." Otherwise, how can I expect them to trust me and know how much I really love and care about them? They won't tell me what's happening in their lives if I don't tell them what's happening in mine, especially if they find out from someone else. Wonder if they would understand why I feel it best for them that I not write all these things now? I go round and round with this decision. I want to tell them, but don't think I should! So, for now and perhaps until I'm well enough to go to California and talk to them, I'll not try to put it in a letter. It will be better to do it in person. I hope that will be soon. Again, it could be six months. I miss them very much, but it would be unwise right now for them to visit me or for me to fly there. I just want them to be well and happy.

The pictures Elly sent you were just ones that in my "fog" I thought you might want. The little girl in the picture is my girlfriend's grand-daughter, in case you were wondering!

I just meant to write a short note! Hope you can read this scribble. Thanks again for everything. I worry about my family a lot and hope everything is going as well as the letters indicate. I'm reassured that you're there to keep me posted.

Kiss the girls for me, and give them and Fred my love.

Take care of yourself—please!

I love you.

Bev

I cried as I finished reading the letter. I had so much to forget, but did I want to forget as much as forgive? I needed to absolve the many doctors and myself. The past could serve as a foundation for the future if I let it work for me, not against me. Look on it as experiences that made you a stronger and hopefully wiser person, I contemplated. You have so much in your life now. Maybe it took all that's happened to get to this point of contentment, to realize your priorities, to know what is important. You now have a chance to do what's important to you, not what the rest of the world wants you to do. *No,* you mustn't forget the past; you just won't live in it anymore. You'll live in the present, in today—that's all you really have anyway.

"Enjoy," my Grandma would have said.

"I'll try, Grandma dear," I whispered.

6
Searching for Answers

The next day I evaluated my problems to see what further steps could be taken to solve them.

"Don't stay in the problem too long," Susan advised. "Get into the solution."

"I know sometimes I spend too much time thinking about the problem or looking for the perfect solution. Then my thoughts go 'round and 'round and I get nothing done. All I get out of it is a giant headache!"

"Everyone's like that sometimes. We just have to select the most likely solution and act upon it, then get on with our lives, leaving the results to God. Have faith that the results will be as they are intended to be."

"And if there's nothing I can do about the situation, accept it and go on with the business of living."

"Yes, and remember, no one's perfect. So take action and put those problems in your past."

"Hey, that's a good key word!"

"What word?"

"PAST. That word. P stands for the problem and so on. A for action. No, let's make that the answers I'm going to write down. Then S for start to take action and T . . ."

"T is for trust in God!" Susan added.

"Great! Problem, Answer, Start, Trust spells PAST. Another item to put on my refrigerator, as a reminder for me to get out of the problem and into the solution."

"Very clever! Problem, Answer, Start and Trust. I'll have to remember that."

"Now the biggies for me are not being able to accept my illness and feeling guilty when I have to say 'no.' I lie about my health, to others as well as myself, and then I overdo. It's like I'm being impelled to move even when I'm near exhaustion. 'Keep moving, keep moving,' my head says, until I drop. Acceptance is the key, I think, to all of this. Acceptance of myself, my illness, my limitations, my good qualities too, everything. Acceptance of everything!

"When I can do this, really feel the acceptance inside, then I'll be able to reduce the anger I feel."

"And don't feel guilty about having all this anger. I read that feeling anger is a characteristic phase which one goes through when diagnosed with lupus. Or with any chronic incurable disease for that matter. Stifling your feelings is unhealthy, so don't keep them a secret. Share them. And, of course, loving acceptance of yourself, your body and your capabilities, as you said, is the key, the answer."

Susan was right. Ever since my illness had begun, I had kept my anger inside, under tight control, wearing a smile when I felt like exploding. Mostly my rage was directed at the pain that traveled through my body, and the never-ending fatigue. Another thing I didn't know at that time was that the irritability I suffered also stemmed from lupus. When you have chronic pain, you have to deal with irritability.

One day I heard an old saying, "The good die young," discussed on television. The "good" keep their hurts inside until the stress explodes into disease and they die. I no longer wanted to die, so I became determined to let my anger out. But how to start?

"Begin by talking honestly to yourself," I recalled hearing on the show. Then I was to take tiny steps toward being candid about my feelings with a close friend, they had said, then with more friends, and soon it would become natural for me to express my feelings. I'd give it a try.

No one will care if you blow up now and then, I lectured to myself. And if they do, so what? You have to do this for yourself. Remember you're only human, so stop expecting perfection. Stop trying to be perfect!

So, with my irritability and emotional rage unleashed, I exploded at my friends over little things, and then I would suffer tremendous guilt and remorse. At the other end of the emotional scale were the tears that burst forth without any apparent reason. My emotions were at the surface, ready to explode at the slightest provocation, raw emotions that were new to me. This isn't working, I observed one day. I'm miserable.

These outbursts relieved some of the tension, but I needed to learn to express my feelings appropriately and to replace my negative emotions entirely with a positive, loving attitude. When I finally learned to say "no" lovingly, without guilt, I found a strange thing happened: people didn't mind. They usually understood, and they still loved me or they didn't. The "no" didn't make the difference. Soon I learned to decline invitations without feeling guilty.

The next time Susan and I talked, she asked, "Well, how are you doing? Expressing yourself? Saying 'no' without feeling guilty?" We laughed at her questions. "And how's the quest for perfection?"

"Okay, okay, enough!" I interrupted, finally getting my giggles under control. "I'm trying. Like you said, no one, nothing is perfect. Except you and me of course!"

Susan had helped me realize that I'd been harder on myself, more demanding of myself than any one else had ever been. And that had to stop if I wanted to feel better.

"Even with the limitations lupus imposes, you can

lead a productive, quality life," Susan said. "Maybe not produce the quantity of work you used to, but so what! You have to learn to slow down. You're 'type A' personality; most people with lupus are. You're ambitious, competitive, a perfectionist. In your case, even your name, 'Beverly' means ambitious. Did you know that?"

"Yes. I read that somewhere, but it also means peace and harmony. I used to think that meant how I should react toward the whole world, ignoring the turmoil that went on inside. Now I'm aiming for the peace and harmony inside. And I'm getting better on the ambitious drive-myself thing. I really have learned to slow down a little."

"I remember," she said, laughing at the image, "when I first met you. You were always doing three things at the same time, always going at full speed."

"I know what you mean. My daughter and I were talking about that the other day. She reminded me that when she was ten years old, I attended the university full time, worked full time, and took care of the house, all while raising three children. I always went, as you said, full speed ahead. I still have trouble slowing down. Parks recently said that I do more work than most well people he knows. He too suggested that I try slowing down. 'You know, smell the roses along the way.' I never learned how to do that when there's so much to do."

"Make the time! Work out a schedule, one that's best for you. And remember, pacing yourself is nothing to feel guilty about. When you take care of yourself, your family and friends benefit also. Then you can be there for them, but your needs have to come first or you can't do for anyone. Also, put some fun in your life. I used to push myself so hard, I didn't have time to think."

"That's true for me, too. I couldn't stop! Working

full speed kept me from enjoying everyday living. If I can work out a schedule as you suggest, I won't have to do that anymore. My mind can be more relaxed, more serene. I can put more fun in my life, and it's about time!"

"And pacing yourself will mean fewer hospitalizations," my friend reminded me.

"I'm all for that! Now, how about this being alone. Most of the time, I can accept the pain and weakness, but not the loneliness. This seems to be one of my greatest problems right now."

"Expand your friendships," Susan suggested. "I've heard you talk about Steve, and of your friend Parks and others. Maybe now it's time to put some new friends in your life, the people from the rap groups."

I desperately wanted people in my life who understood. That was the key word with me, for even with a loving family and friends, I still felt alone. That horrifying, depressing loneliness that made me feel so empty inside.

"I've often felt as if I were on a desert island all by myself," I said.

"Lupus is bad enough, but it's especially difficult when you live alone, like you do. Putting more friends in your life might be the answer. There are people who really understand how you feel—they've had to endure the same disease. Keep in touch with them. Not only can you draw on their experiences, you can also help others. That's what support groups are for. You told me that in the group, you share your experiences, strengths and hopes and help each other. See more of these people. You don't ever have to feel alone again."

I'd heard those words before and knew them to be true. It had worked for me in regard to alcohol and drugs, and it would work with lupus too.

So call I did, most frequently to Laura, my first

contact with the rap groups. We became fast friends. We laughed and cried together and shared daily happenings as well as our experiences with doctors and lupus. We discussed our similar past symptoms, the failure of doctors to diagnose us, and the fact that we had both been called hypochondriacs.

"It's all in your head" was a familiar phrase we had both heard often.

"Then one time," Laura recounted, "I happened to go to a doctor when I had a rash across the bridge of my nose and below my eyes, roughly in the shape of a butterfly. The nose rash resembled its body and the rash on my cheeks below my eyes looked like its wings. We're now familiar with this as the 'butterfly rash.' But then I didn't know what it was. There were many times over the years before I was diagnosed that I had this rash, but didn't go to a doctor, so an important clue wasn't presented. The dermatologist who finally saw the rash sent me to a rheumatologist and the diagnosis was made."

"So you have discoid LE too."

"Yes. Some people have this kind only, some have the internal type, systemic LE, and some have both, like I do."

"I didn't get the rash," I said. "That made it difficult to diagnose. No one even looked for lupus until I went to a rheumatologist here in California. Actually, even though I'd been referred to over thirty different doctors and specialists, a rheumatologist was not among them. It was only after years of illness that a physical therapist finally suggested it."

"That's one of the problems. People don't get to the proper specialists," Laura confirmed. "And even then, it's a difficult disease to diagnose. The symptoms are many, and varied, and intermittent, and can be symptoms of other diseases besides lupus."

"I read somewhere that there are only a few

hundred symptoms of illnesses, but many thousands of different diseases that could cause those symptoms."

"And lupus has so many different symptoms it mimics many other diseases. It's often called the "great imitator." Some of the mistaken diagnoses have been inner ear infections, flu, poison ivy, sunstroke, syphilis, epilepsy, anemia, virus infection, heart disease, kidney disease, and emotional problems. The list is almost endless."

"I had many of those. Several times before my diagnosis, I vowed to never, NEVER see another doctor, but those resolutions were always broken. I felt that I was grasping at straws when I did go again, but I would get so desperate, so sick. What else could I do?"

"Well," Laura reiterated, "the main trouble was that we weren't being sent to the right kind of doctor."

"Oh, I almost forgot," I said. "Do you have the criteria for lupus? I have to send someone a copy, and I can't find mine anywhere."

"Hold on a minute. I'll look."

Laura went to find the list and I searched for a pen and paper; neither were ever around when I wanted them!

"Found it," Laura said. "There are eleven items listed. It says if a person has four or more, a doctor's advice should be sought to determine if one actually has lupus. Do you want me to read them to you?"

"Yes, but go slow, so I can write them down."

Laura read:

"1. The butterfly rash we were talking about.
2. Disc-shaped sores, usually on the face, arms or chest. This is discoid lupus.
3. Sensitivity to sun exposure.
4. Mouth sores, often in the roof of the mouth.
5. Arthritis.
6. Kidney trouble, protein in the urine.

7. Neurological trouble, seizures or psychosis.
8. Pericarditis or pleuritis.
9. Anemia or low blood count.
10. False-positive syphilis test or positive ANA test results.
11. Positive results on any of the other blood tests for SLE."

"I also had fatigue, pain, weakness and other symptoms of lupus that are not on that list."

"Right," Laura agreed. "I had those symptoms, too, but for diagnostic purposes, this is the criteria the American Rheumatism Association established recently. Now, after ruling out rheumatoid arthritis, scleroderma and polymyositis, a diagnosis of systemic lupus can be made if, as I said, four or more of the eleven criteria are met. Like most people with the disease, you and I have had many of the subjective symptoms of lupus. Pain, weakness, tiring easily, loss of energy, and generalized aching are common ones."

"It's a lot to accept," I said.

"Well, we have to adjust our lives and do the best we can to make things easier for ourselves, yet not become lupus cripples."

"What's that?" I asked.

"A lupus cripple is someone who would say, for example, 'I can't go to the Hollywood Bowl because I can't walk from the parking lot and up the stairs.' A lupus survivor would make arrangements to be dropped off in front with no apology necessary. We don't think of ourselves as frail freaks. Instead, we're hothouse orchids that just need special handling."

"I'll have to remember that."

"Of course, there are days when I'm too tired to move," she continued. "I'm not speaking of ordinary tiredness due to lack of rest or from healthy physical activity. I'm talking about a fatigue and exhaustion that hits every inch of your body—the type where you haven't the strength to lift your head off your pillow, nor the energy to hold a toothbrush to brush your teeth."

"Boy, Laura, I really relate to that!" I said. "There are so many days that my energy level is so extremely low, my body feels as if it weighs a ton. I can hardly breathe, let alone drag myself out of bed. It's the kind of fatigue you described. I tried to explain that to a doctor once, but he didn't understand. And sometimes I feel nervous and restless, especially my head. When an attack of fatigue comes, I guess I need to learn to relax. Sounds easy—wonder why it's not! And how do I explain it to others!"

"I know it's hard, but you learn not to explain or make excuses. Your responsibility is to take care of yourself. I had to eliminate some people from my life, and you may have to also. With family it's a little more difficult, but not impossible. As I said, your first responsibility is to yourself, to take care of yourself. If you don't do that, you may not be around to have family or friends. Or at the very least, you'll suffer for it."

"Makes sense," I said. "Still, it's hard for me to say 'no.' It sounds easy, and I don't know why I can't do it. I have this very demanding boss—*myself!* No one else pushes me. I've really been blessed with an understanding family and great friends, but I've found it difficult not to be able to respond to people as I could in the past. However, I'm getting better. I've also come to realize that I've experienced enough criticism in my life—now I need to be with loving, non-critical people so I can express my feelings without receiving negative vibes. I can't maintain a positive attitude with negative people in my life."

"I think you're doing great. You're honest, open-minded, and you are willing to do whatever is necessary to improve the quality of your life. And you're a very loving person. You'll make it! I know you will."

"Thanks," I responded. "I needed to hear that. Say, are you going to the rap session across town? I understand it's a new group."

"That's tomorrow, isn't it? No, I won't be able to make it, maybe the next one. Now we'd better hang up and get some of that rest we keep talking about!"

"Pace ourselves!" we said in unison.

One o'clock the next day came quickly. I rushed out the door to get to the lupus rap group. Remember when you didn't even want to go—now you're eager to get there. I smiled to myself.

7
Lupus Self-help Session

A typical lupus rap session consisted of six to twelve people, ranging from the newly-diagnosed to those who had been treated for years. Some spoke freely, others were shy. When I arrived the meeting was about to begin.

As I walked into the room, I heard the familiar laughter that had surprised and captivated me at other meetings. We were certainly a happy group in spite of this terrible disease. Dianne, a lupus patient herself, was leading today's session, and when I settled in a chair, she began sharing her story.

"I wasn't diagnosed until 1980, after about twenty years of illness. I'm not talking about illness every single day of my life—I had remissions and flares—but it probably started when I was seventeen years old. At that time, I lost a tremendous amount of weight and I was very tired. I hurt all over, but I had no really specific complaint. I went through a great deal of testing, but the doctors didn't know what was wrong with me. I was tested for everything from leukemia to diabetes, and they really didn't come up with anything, except for that era's disease of the decade. It was hypoglycemia. So they told me to eat better, take better care of myself, and for no reason at all, I happened to get better. But lupus can be that way; you can go into remission without making any change in your life.

"And then, at various times, I would become extremely tired and have aches and pains, but that would last only a short time. Just vague symptoms that came and went. But in the seventies, my condition worsened. In 1974 I walked through a sliding glass door, and I thought some of the glass had been left in me because of the pains in my hands. At the same time, I was being treated for what the doctors diagnosed as an allergic reaction on my back. I was also sent to an orthopedic surgeon for pain in my knee. He wanted to operate but I refused. Again I began to lose weight and was told to eat more. I became incredibly fatigued. The doctor told me, 'Well, you know, women who stay at home with little toddlers suffer stress . . . you just need to rest more. You'll be fine. If you like I'll give you some tranquilizers.' "

"That's what happened to me," Claire chimed in. "I started taking the tranquilizer Librium. My marriage crumbled and a psychiatrist was recommended. Was your marriage affected by all that?"

"Yes," Dianne said. "It was difficult. I was always tired, too tired to keep up with everything. Meals became catch-as-catch-can because I was just too tired to shop and cook and take care of my family. It was also an emotional time. I felt ill and the doctors found nothing. Different symptoms were being treated by different specialists without them ever getting together. I had inflammation underneath my fingernails and they were treating me for a fungus infection, forcing fungicide under my nails—very painful. The one thing they did that helped was to inject cortisone into the sore bumps on my fingers. That was helping. For the allergy, a rash that was on my back . . ."

"Oh, you had discoid also?" Claire asked.

"Yes," Dianne said. "And the rash was taped with

cortisone cream with saran wrap all over my back!"

"Didn't they ever send you to a dermatologist?"

"It was a dermatologist who was doing that! He was the same doctor who was forcing fungicide under my fingernails and injecting the shots of cortisone into the little lumps that were all over my hands. At the same time I had swollen lymph nodes. I was sent to an ear, nose and throat doctor, and he didn't know what was wrong. He suggested that I eat more."

"How awful! How did you feel with all that going on and nothing being detected?"

"I just knew in my heart that something was wrong, but I didn't know what. I started questioning my own sanity at that point, because after going to all those doctors and spending all that money, they couldn't find anything wrong with me. So it must be in my head. Finally, after many years, I stopped going to doctors. I wasn't going to have my legs operated on, so I gave up on seeking a diagnosis. Later I went to another dermatologist for a completely unrelated problem. He suspected lupus, although he didn't tell me his misgivings. I asked him about a rash that kept appearing, and he suggested that I take a blood test. This doctor is pretty dumb, I thought. I have a rash and he wants to draw blood! For an allergy!

"He also wanted a biopsy. Finally after all this, he told me that I had systemic lupus erythematosus. All I could understand amidst those big words, was the name lupus."

"I'd never heard of the disease when I was diagnosed," I said. "Had you?"

"No. I went to the library and scared myself to death! 'ninety percent death rate in first five years!' No, this could not be me! There was no way in the world that it could be me. By the time I finished reading about lupus, I was in a total state of shock."

"I felt relieved when they finally diagnosed me,"

Claire said. "At least I *had* something! I wasn't going crazy, and it wasn't all in my mind!

"I was relieved that there was something wrong with me, but I wasn't prepared for what it was. The disease frightened me so much that I couldn't enjoy the relief. Still, it released me from all the doubts and the self-recrimination that maybe I was just a lazy person, that maybe I was no good. It relieved me enough so I could carry on with my life.

"Before I was diagnosed, I questioned my sanity. Afterwards I thought 'This can't be happening to me.' Then I learned about a book, *Lupus, the Body Against Itself*, by Dr. Sheldon Paul Blau. When I had finished reading the book, I felt better, knowing more about the disease. I had been told about the book by a woman whose dog had the disease and her vet had recommended the book. I thought how strange it is that because of her dog, here's a woman who knew more about the disease than I!

"For over a year, my husband denied that I had the disease. 'If you ignore it, it'll go away,' he would say. 'How do you know you have it, how do the doctors know? Maybe they're wrong.' But I wanted that diagnosis. I didn't want to be crazy!"

"Boy, I know what you mean," June chimed in. "But the lupus group helped me. I felt less different, and it helped to talk to people on the hot line. 'Hey, you're not crazy' I would tell myself. I learned from others' experiences, and I learned to explain to my husband what was going on with me.

"Some days I feel good and I don't want any help from anyone. Other days, I really need that extra help. It's hard to get a balance. Now if I'm not feeling well and I need help, I'll tell my family, otherwise they let me alone to do my own thing. That's how we're able to handle it now, but it was hard in the beginning."

"At first I felt tremendous relief," I said, "but when I

realized that this was not going to go away, that it was incurable and chronic, I exploded with terrible anger. I still have some anger left that I have to work through. It comes out, especially when I'm in a flare."

"Oh yeah! I did too," said Terry, a young man in his early thirties. "When they diagnosed me, I was really mad, mostly at all the pressure from my family. And then when the doctor gave me steroids I got violent. I began throwing things. I went through a lot of stages, and eventually it seemed as if I would level out, but then they put me on a higher dose when I went into the hospital. I hallucinated, and my emotions went haywire. When I went into the hospital, I had a good attitude, but I lost control of my mind as a result of the drugs. I was doped up on twelve different pills when the doctors told me that I would have to go on dialysis. I thought I had accepted it, and then came the anger; and when I got rid of that, then the drugs made me depressed. I went from three months of not sleeping to massive depression. I've never been as scared as I was then. Sometimes I think that the drugs are more scary than the disease itself."

"I remember you calling me," Dianne said, "because I had a similar experience with my family."

"Yes, I would call and ask how long all this was going to take. I was boggled by all the emotions."

"You were married when they diagnosed you?"

"Yes, but talking to my family wasn't the same as talking to someone who'd had similar experiences. My wife and my parents went to a couple of lupus meetings, but then they weren't interested in going anymore. I'm glad I had someone to call. It kept me focused on the fact that I'm not insane, I'm not losing my mind. It is normal to go through all these stages. I hear everyone talk about the emotions, and it helps me cope, gives me peace of mind. I don't feel the fear any more, and it helps the anger. My dad also helps.

He believes in laughing a lot, and laughter helps me to cope."

"I think laughter saved my life," I said. "I like to laugh, and I try to be around people who have a happy outlook. I read that laughter reduces stress and relieves a person of tension, and I believe it. Anyway, it surely does for me—relaxes my body, clears my head, and makes me feel better. It's like a nice hug! And that's one of the great things about these meetings. We can all laugh together. By the way, Terry, did you have a lot of problems before you were diagnosed? What was it like then?"

"I got burned out and couldn't hold a job. I'd get moody and incredibly tired, and I didn't have a long steady flow of energy. I used to have back problems that turned out to be my kidneys trying to tell me something, like I was getting overloaded. I tried to eat more to get more energy, but no matter how much I consumed, it didn't make any difference. I would be dragging while all my friends that were my age were plugging right along. Then one day I got sunburned and was taken into emergency, but the doctors couldn't find the problem.

"The next day, I went to our family doctor and he discovered blood in my urine. He got so excited that it scared me. I didn't think doctors were supposed to get that upset.

"From there I was referred to a surgeon and then to an internist, and it was this doctor who made the diagnosis."

"Did you feel relieved or angry?"

"Oh, what a relief it was," he said with a laugh. "It wasn't in my head; it was actually happening! But then I couldn't get my energy back. You know, I like to work. I'm a clean person and I like everything just so—I'm particular about things. But now I have to slow down. I used to go until I couldn't move any more. It's mentally hard on me, especially as a young person. At one point I felt neurotic. I was losing all my self-esteem."

"I imagine being male makes it even more difficult," Dianne interjected. "And trying to earn a living and everything."

"Right," he said. "Trying to be a provider. One of the things that hurt me the most was not being able to go surfing. That's just really hard on me, and I still have dreams about doing that. Going out on the water meant a lot to me. That was my big escape. I'd been doing it for twelve years, and my work was making surf boards. I used to be a skinny blond—now I'm a dark-haired pudgy guy. It's hard."

"Did all the steroids do that?"

"Yes, they also darkened my hair."

"Age does that too!" Dianne giggled. We all laughed with her.

"You had to throw that in," he groaned good-naturedly. "I always thought that age lightened it! You know, gray hair and all that stuff."

"True. Actually the sun probably lightened your hair, and then when you couldn't be in the sun . . ."

"Do steroids really darken your hair?"

"It took all the gray out of my hair."

"It took all my hair!"

"It took all your hair! Really!"

"Yes."

"Boy, that's all I need!"

"I'm in total remission now, but I still have weakness and pain. It never goes away, even in remission."

"The main thing with me, I think, is being a male," Terry said, "and being the provider. That's really hard. Sometimes I'd just rather die because I want to do more, but I can't. I've lost my freedom. When you have an illness and lose your mind and your health, what do you do then? People are always saying that they lost this and that, but at least they have their health. What do you do when you lose that?

"You've come a long way, Terry. I remember when you first came here. You're a lot more stable now. You were totally downhill for a long time, but now you can see some light at the end of the tunnel."

"Yes, I'm more stable now, but it's taken so long."

"It's different for everyone," Dianne explained. "You have to work through certain stages, and no one stays in the same stage. You're going to hit anger. You're going to hit depression, denial. Everyone goes back and forth through these stages. The best we can hope for is to hold onto the acceptance stage for longer periods of time. But you know, if someone is depressed and feels like crying, I say, 'go ahead.' You deserve it. Why not? Don't feel guilty about being depressed. A good cry does a lot of good sometimes. It tends to shorten my depression or anger stages.

"I talk with a lot of people on the Lupus Hotline, and I give people permission to cry. Some people think it is wrong; they think they have to be a Pollyanna all the time, and I just don't feel that we have to. Sometimes if I can say 'I am depressed, I feel like crying,' or if I can verbally work through some of my problems, it seems to help. And it's okay. You have a right to be depressed. You hurt. You feel bad. You're dependent on something—you have to take these medications. But it's okay. I'm going to be okay and so are you. Just know that you're not alone."

"I think that what you said is really true. I went through a denial of the disease, but I also went through a big denial of what I was feeling because I thought it was wrong to feel that way."

"But it's not wrong."

"Right. And the other thing is that while it's okay that I'm feeling that way now, I try not to hang on to the negative feelings. Those have to change. They're not going to stay with me. For me, there's a danger if I hang onto anger or depression too long. I think that a big part of accepting . . ."

"Yes, that's the key word. Everything is accepting—that it's okay to feel angry. I'm not perfect. I don't know what makes me feel I have to be perfect!"

"I just want to make a comment about depression," Terry said. "I was deceived about depression. After I got out of the hospital, I felt suicidal because of the chemicals I had to take. There's a difference between chemical depression and other depression. I wanted to hang onto my wife and never let her go, and the doctor told me not to walk down the block by myself. I was like an old man. I had lost thirty pounds; I was all shriveled up, couldn't walk without a cane, and everyone stared at me, unable to believe how I looked. That was scary. It was mental torture. My mind was trapped in a body that used to move around and all of a sudden wasn't moving anymore. At the end of the week, I had progressed to a wheelchair, but I couldn't handle the chair too well and that didn't do my self-image any good.

"Also, it's amazing how people look at you in a wheelchair. I was in one a couple of times when my feet became so inflamed I couldn't walk, and just my being visibly disabled made people uncomfortable. We may all be disabled, but we look fine. Our symptoms are somewhat invisible to most, but being in a wheelchair where the world is standing and you're sitting, and you're being pushed around, is a whole different perspective on life. I certainly had a different perspective after being in one for just a short time. It was enough to shock me. Most of the time people would talk to whoever was accompanying me rather than talking to me directly, as though I were a non-person. Having a visible handicap is different from having an invisible one. People don't think you're sick when you look well, and that causes problems too. But with a visible handicap, it's an entirely different set of problems."

"Yes, people are always saying to me, 'you look fine,' and I simply say 'thank you.' "

"That's hard to live with. Like, the patient looked fine, but he died," Terry said. We all laughed along with him.

That was the thing that impressed me. We laughed at ourselves and the situation. Somehow it lightened the load. We all had serious health problems, but everyone could find some humor in the situation.

"Yes—or sometimes if I feel like being totally honest and a friend says 'you look fine,' I say 'thank you, I feel rotten!' But only with people I know."

"It depends on how comfortable you are. I generally just say 'thank you.' "

"Yes, and I feel rotten!" We all laughed.

"My family knows better than to say that to me. They know why I'm on the couch, and it's not because I feel fine."

"Right. And on the serious side, I don't think people mean anything by the comment. So I choose not to take offense at it and just thank them. Besides, most people don't want to know any more."

"Sometimes it's hard when I go to church," Terry confided. "The older men are still feisty, they haven't been through what I have, and they have all kinds of ideas about what I should be doing. 'Come on, just keep busy,' they'll say. 'You'll feel better.' And I'm sitting there in tremendous pain saying to myself, 'Don't let it bug you. They just don't know.' What can you do? I try to explain it a little bit, and it just goes in one ear and out the other."

"Right, especially because most people have never heard of this disease. So then I have to try to explain it, and they just don't understand it."

"How do you explain it?"

"Well, it depends on the experience of the person asking. Often it's easier for me to just say it's in the family of arthritis, of rheumatoid arthritis, depending on who's asking the question. Do they really want to know?"

"I guess what they're asking is, 'How does it affect you? What are your symptoms?' "

"I say that I'm allergic to my own body," Terry said.

"And that's true!"

"And," Terry continued, "I've got the opposite of AIDS. My system is beating me up, while AIDS victims' systems are not doing a thing and they're dying from it. I get funny about it. I feel as long as there's life, there's hope."

"People are working to find a cure, and I think it'll happen in the next five years."

"Right on."

"And in the meantime, we can learn to live with it."

"We're all going to die someday, anyway. It's how we live that counts. And even with lupus, I can have a quality life. It just takes a little work on my part."

"But when you're young, it's hard to see your life going so fast. In one year, my body went through more trauma than most people have in eighty years. Everything came crashing down. I was cornered with this disease. I'm crammed in with pressure and stress and illness, so I go through all these ups and downs trying to cope."

"If you had been one hundred percent alone, you might not have made it."

"True, if it hadn't been for the talk groups . . ."

"If I didn't have somebody to talk to—a support system within my own family or friends—I don't know how I would have coped."

"It's not that I want sympathy. . . "

"No, all I want is understanding."

"Right," we all said in unison.

"Claire, maybe, as a nurse, you can answer this. I heard that depression is a manifestation of lupus. Is that true?"

"Can be," Claire responded. She was a retired nurse and a lupus patient. "It's very difficult to say which comes first, the chicken or the egg. It can be a symptom of lupus, but having a chronic disease, in itself, can make you depressed and suicidal. So it's a complicated procedure to find out whether it's clinical or not."

"You mentioned being suicidal. I've gotten that way, quite recently, as a matter of fact. But it passes, if I just hang in there. However, I understand the feelings Terry had. It's very painful."

"Not to change the subject, but what did you mean by 'manifestation'? How it appears . . .? "

"Right. When do we cross the bridge from lupus to depression? Does lupus make depression?"

"It can. Just as you can have a kidney problem caused by the disease."

"Lupus can also produce memory loss. This is very common, especially the short-term memory loss."

"Boy, that's for sure! But in any chronic disease, like you said, you can end up in a depression."

"But if you ask, can lupus do it, I say 'yes' to whatever you're asking. Anything you ask, lupus can do. It can make you go blind, lose your hair, make your feet hurt so bad you can't walk . . ."

"It can attack any part of the body, so why not."

"It'll even attack the vocal cords."

"But remember, just because lupus *can* do it doesn't mean it will. Every case is different. What happens to you won't necessarily happen to me. My disease is my disease, and yours is yours."

"I don't want yours!"

"And I don't want yours, either!" We all cracked up at that.

"But, I think the feelings we experience are similar."

"Right, that's one thing we have in common."

"Frustration, for one. The worse thing of all is that I never know when I get up in the morning how I'm going to feel."

"And boy, that's depressing. Or I wake up in the morning feeling okay and by afternoon . . ."

Everyone started talking at once, in agreement.

"You make an appointment and you can't keep it. It's devastating not knowing from hour to hour what will strike you next or where."

"Right, I never know."

"We used to have a baby sitter who loved working for us. We'd make plans, and come evening, I'd be too tired to go out for dinner. And that's the epitome! We'd have to cancel, but she got paid anyway. And this would happen quite often."

"This is so amazing. It happens to me too, and people don't understand how I can be too tired to throw some clothes on and go out to eat. They were trying to do something nice for me, and they couldn't understand that I just didn't have the energy to get dressed. My parents in their eighties have more energy than I have."

"The disease takes it all. That's something I've had to learn to accept. For example, I don't go out at night. Most people know that I don't go out at night, and that's how it is."

"It's worse in the beginning when you're used to leading an active life and suddenly you're struck with this mysterious disease that prevents you from doing so many things."

"Well, being older," said Claire, "I don't anticipate as much in life, perhaps, as the younger people do. I realize that I will become less active; I will have less opportunity to take part in things. It doesn't bother me so much anymore, but it did when I was leading an active life. That was really hard to give up. It really did bother me then."

"Let me tell you something about Claire," Dianne said, smiling warmly at the nurse. "She had a 50th reunion of her nursing school class which she couldn't attend. She had planned on that for two years. Then the day before she planned to leave, she got pneumonia. So, you see, no matter what your age, it doesn't mean that disappointments don't happen that you have no control over. Claire's just being modest."

"Well . . ." Claire laughed. "But maybe I've just learned to accept it better, and that's part of learning to live with the disease."

"As a nurse, had you heard of the disease?"

"Yes, but most of my experience was with the young child-bearing woman. So often, their disease was apt to be more profound, and their episodes fatal. So that was my experience. You see, I was sixty-six years old before I really became ill with lupus, even though I had had it off and on all my life. Now I know that I had rheumatic fever when I was nineteen. Five months later I had a severe attack of dryness in spots all over my entire body. I just woke up one morning and I was all swollen. I was put to bed, but I couldn't stand to have anything touching me. I itched all over. It was very puzzling to the doctors; they didn't understand what it was all about. One morning five days later, I began menstruating, so the doctors chalked it up as a premenstrual problem of some sort. There were other incidents like this, and then in my thirties I began to have weekly incidents of extreme fatigue. Raising a family, it became a serious problem. I couldn't do all the things I wanted to do. But then it went away. I had three normal children, no problems with my pregnancies. So I know I was in long periods of remission and there was never a need to seek a diagnosis."

"So how were you diagnosed?"

"That was kind of odd. I first became ill in 1978, in Hawaii, just like Beverly. I was in the process of moving back to California, retiring from nursing, when I was hospitalized for extremely severe pain all over my body. I couldn't stand to be touched. My right leg wouldn't function, and I was in a walker. My back was bad for five months. Finally, in December, I was able to make the move. Here in California, I talked to a doctor who suspected the disease, but for some reason did not want to tell me. So for one year, I had treatments for osteoarthritis, and it wasn't until a year later I found out that I had another kind of arthritis that, even as a nurse, I had never heard of before. It was called palindromic."

"What's that?" several voices questioned.

"That's what I asked! I found out that the term simply means recurring. Well, I knew something was recurring—I didn't have to go to the doctor to find that out!

"Then, the following year, I applied for health insurance. It was during the examination, when I was rejected, that I really found out. The insurance application came back, and I read that I had been rejected because of having been under treatment for lupus!"

"I'm not able to get medical insurance either,"

"Neither am I."

"This is a real problem. Medical bills can be extensive."

"That was a heck of a way to find out your diagnosis!"

"That's the way I found it out," Claire continued. "The doctors didn't tell me, but they had to tell the insurance company."

"Before I forget, I want to mention that these rap groups have been very good for my husband too."

"My husband never went to a rap group, but I've heard that it can be very helpful."

"Yes, he could hear what some of the other women were saying, and it helped him to understand me better. Except for today, he's attended almost every meeting I've gone to. He wants to understand what's going on with me, and then he can better cope with it all."

"If you have lupus, and your spouse denies it, then you're on your own. And it's really hard."

"I was lucky to have a daughter who understood. So many children don't want to hear that Mommy can't do this, that or the next thing. Normal children tend to be a little selfish. I was very lucky. We explained to her right away that I had something, and that things were going to be happening to me that would necessitate her helping out occasionally, that I wouldn't be able to do some of the things that the other mothers were doing."

"But it was great that your daughter knew and was able to accept it."

"Yes, she did quite well handling the news. I didn't get the feedback that a lot of parents get from their children—they don't want to hear about it. They complain when Mom can't do everything. So, I've been very lucky."

"I had the disease while my children were growing up, living at home, but it was undiagnosed. So the times my body gave out were always called other things, mostly ending up with an emotional angle. It was horrible when I would feel so ill and not know why. The doctors gave me a lot of medication to help but never, of course, got to the root of the problem. They didn't even look for the disease, even though I had all the classic symptoms. I guess I still have some anger about that. Mostly because of my family and all that I missed and all that I wasn't able to do for and with them. The periodic fatigue was so bad and so indescribable. Even now, I have trouble describing it."

"Everyone does. Sometimes I think only someone with this disease can really understand lupus fatigue."

"That's descriptive. Lupus fatigue! It really is different from other fatigue."

"Right," Dianne said with a smile. "And now we'd better close this meeting so we don't all get it!"

The meeting ended with the same laughter that I had heard at the beginning. And I felt great!

8

Research on Lupus

With each lupus flare something would come into my life that helped me improve its quality. For example, I knew that stress, or rather distress, was an important factor in triggering flares for me. After one such flare, Laura sent me an excellent article on stress that put much of what I already knew into perspective. I thought it would make a good acronym and telephoned Parks to tell him about it.

"Remember the acronym HALT that I have on my refrigerator door?" I asked. "It reminds me that I shouldn't get too **H**ungry, **A**ngry, **L**onely or **T**ired? Well, Laura sent me a wonderful article on stress by Jean Scott and I thought that an acronym could be written on the points involved in the article. I wanted to get your opinion."

"Why don't you read it to me?"

"Okay, but it's long . . ."

"That's all right."

"Well, here goes:"

STRESS[1]
by Jean Scott

Stress is one of the big causes of "flare-ups" for the lupus person. It would take a large book to list all the reasons why they feel so much stress, but a few of them might be:

---

[1]. Jean Scott, "Stress," Minnesota News & Notes, No. 3, February 1977

1. Lupus people feel a great deal of anxiety and sometimes a feeling of panic, either from symptoms they are now having or the constant worry that new symptoms may develop.
2. Many lupus patients feel almost constant fatigue, and often this is made worse because their sleep is interrupted several times during the night due to the pain.
3. Most lupus people worry about their health, which causes more stress. This is especially true for those who must hold down jobs. They constantly worry about not being able to feel well enough to go to work, yet are afraid to miss too much work for fear of losing their jobs.
4. Lupus people know they must get enough rest; yet, especially, if they find it difficult to accept their illness, they may become tense and restless and unable to relax when they are resting. This is further complicated by guilt feelings, especially if they have a family and are in charge of the house and feel they should be up to cooking, sewing, doing laundry or other household tasks.
5. Lupus people often take another person's comments personally. One comment they may hear often is, "but you look so well." This can be hard to accept if one really feels sick inside. Lupus education can do much to correct this.
6. Lupus people often feel remote from other people and things they used to like—family, friends, sports, books. This also creates guilt feelings—and consequently more stress.
7. Another thing that creates stress for many lupus people is that they're not feeling happy about their personal appearance—maybe the face is blotchy with discoid lesions or butterfly rash; they may have swelling from cortisone or fluid retention which makes them feel fat, so that they may not even do the things they could to improve their appearance.
8. A lupus person dreads many everyday situations that others may look forward to—playing with the children, going to parties or even to the store. When lupus people are invited to a party they may accept and look forward to it a great deal. But comes the

day of the party, they may feel very ill or so extremely tired that the party sounds uninviting. How do they explain this to their hostess, or maybe even to their spouses if the spouse has looked forward to the event, especially if the spouse has not yet accepted the patient's illness?

When I think of the famous words of Reinhold Niebuhr, 'God grant me the serenity to accept the things I cannot change, the courage to change the things I can, and the wisdom to know the difference,' I wonder if he might have had the lupus person in mind. Yes, there are so many things that a lupus person must accept, but there are also many positive things we can do to cut down the amount of stress in our lives and thus possibly avoid another flare-up. Below are a few of them.

1. Get enough sleep and rest. Take a daily nap. This is possible even if you are working. Establish a regular time for this. (I use the time when the evening paper is delivered as my regular resting time.) Since rest is *absolutely* essential for the lupus person, do not feel that you have to explain to family and friends; be selfish in this and everyone will benefit in the long run.
2. If your health permits, get regular exercise. Daytime walks may be "Taboo" because of the sun; a walk at dusk as all the lights are coming on in homes is a great time to get your exercise. Relaxed muscles mean relaxed nerves. Tennis, hiking and home or club calisthenics are other exercise possibilities.
3. Avoid hurry, flurry, worry. You might do as Ma Bell suggests—don't run all over town looking for something. 'Let your fingers do the walking.' If necessary, lower your housekeeping standards, possibly only you will notice if the bathroom tile doesn't get washed this week. Many things we worry about never happen.
4. Love more. Most people need to learn to love people and use things, instead of loving things and using people. Love can be as healing as potent drugs.
5. Listen to your body. When you are under stress, you get symptoms of anxiety. Coping with anxiety is like reading a barometer—there is little you can do

about the changes in the weather but you can learn to observe the warning signals and back off, ease up. Let's reverse that old rule and 'put off until tomorrow what we don't feel like doing today.'

6. Don't be afraid of compromise. Seldom is the ideal situation available. In a stressful situation, you can either fight back or compromise.
7. Avoid coping solutions that involve alcohol or tranquilizers. A little relaxation is fine, but drinking or turning to drugs each time you are faced with a problem could lead to addiction.
8. Identify your fears. It might be helpful even to list them. Talk your problems over with your family and other close friends. Try to think of ways to cope with them. Seek information about the things you fear. Knowledge can bring runaway fears down to earth. Dr. Rene Dubois says, 'People can survive and function more easily if they adapt themselves to the peculiarities of each situation. Educational programs will help the lupus person function better whether she is struggling with a job, dealing with her family or adjusting to her illness.'
9. Make decisions, right or wrong, and act upon them. Anxiety or stress results when you sit in the middle and let your indecision tug at you from opposite directions. We must strive to use adult judgement for ourselves as we are usually able to do with ease for a friend or neighbor.
10. Try to laugh more. Laughter is a good tension breaker. Laugh at yourself so that you do not take yourself too seriously.
11. Avoid self-pity. Self-pity is an immature and selfish response to situations and usually a waste of time and energy. Sure, we all go through periods of 'Why me, God?' but this is a waste of energy and time. Live each day and make the most of it. Plutarch said, 'The measure of man's life is not in the length but the well-spending of it.'
12. Avoid loneliness. Reach out; take the initiative in friendship. Seek out compatible people. Join your local lupus group. You can certainly find friendship and support there. This should help erase that 'all alone' feeling that many people talk about.
13. Educate yourself about your illness and then edu-

cate others. Through public awareness and education, funds will be forthcoming for research and possibly a cure for lupus.

14. Take time each day with your personal appearance. There are several good cover-up makeups for covering the butterfly rash. If fluid retention is a problem, look for the stylish caftans and other loose-fitting clothes that conceal, but still look great.
15. Before each visit to your doctor, make a list of questions to ask him and symptoms you want to mention, and thus avoid the stress of 'Why didn't I ask him about . . .' or 'I forgot to tell him about . . .'

IN CONCLUSION: Thales, one of the seven wise men of ancient Greece, was asked what was difficult. He answered, 'To know oneself.' When asked what was easy, he replied, 'To advise another.' You guessed it. I, too, find it hard to avoid stress and get enough rest, but let's all work on it.

"Well, that's it? What do you think?"

"It's great. And I'm sure it could be put into an acronym. Why don't you send it to me. I'll look it over and call you back."

A few days later, Parks telephoned and I asked, "How's it going with the acronym? Do you think we can make one up?"

"Yes."

"Tell me how you do it, so I can help."

"Well, I've done the preliminary work. I wrote down some words that are relevant to the subject, and could be considered as the acronym or part of it. The subject here is STRESS, so that is one possibility. There are so many points involved that we will either need one very long word or several shorter words. Since we are to avoid stress, we could consider as an acronym, STRESS AVOIDANCE, or NO MORE STRESS, or LET'S AVOID STRESS. Probably we could make the acronym using any of these, so I wanted to ask which you prefer."

"I like LET'S AVOID STRESS. It suggests action. What was your choice?"

"I favored that one, too. Now we write down single words that express the points involved in avoiding stress. Then we go again to the thesaurus. . ."

"Hold on, let me get my thesaurus . . . Okay, go ahead."

"Well, for each of the words pertaining to points of stress, we look for synonyms. We get these synonyms so that if we can't express an idea by using a certain word because it doesn't start with one of the letters in the acronym, perhaps one of its synonyms will start with that letter. Get the idea?"

"Yes. Do you already have the groups containing the ideas and their synonyms?"

"Yes. I thought you could help me select words from the groups, one word for each letter of the acronym."

"All right. We start with the letter L. Right?"

"Right. I'll read our choices for this letter and you select one. Okay?"

Using this method, Parks and I made up the words for which the letters of the acronym stood. The next morning I phoned Laura to tell her about it.

"You know that article on stress that you sent me?"

"You mean the one by Jean Scott."

"Yes. It helped me so much that Parks and I decided to make up an acronym to make the points easier to remember. He did most of the work, but I helped a little!"

"Great! Can you read it to me?"

"Sure. There were a lot of good points, so we used a three-word phrase. We called it, LET'S AVOID STRESS:

L — Love more, Laugh more, avoid Loneliness.
E — Educate yourself, with regard to lupus, and pass that education on to others.
T — Tranquilizers and alcohol, avoid them.
S — Sleep (Get plenty).

A — Appearance. Do what you can to improve yourself if the disease has caused rash or fluid retention.
V — Visit your doctor regularly, preferably a rheumatologist. Write out things you want to tell him, questions you want to ask him.
O — Open-mindedness. Offer to negotiate, either with yourself or others. Half a loaf is better than none.
I — Identify your fears.
D — Decisions. Make them to the best of your ability. You know the feeling of relief in your mind when that has been done.

S — Slow down. Avoid hurry, flurry, worry and fury.
T — Tune-in on your body. Stop when you have just a slight feeling of fatigue. Don't wait until you are all knocked out.
R — Rest and Relaxation. Get plenty during the day. Take an afternoon nap.
E — Exercise. Have your rheumatologist advise you on this.
S — Self-pity, avoid it! Surely you know of others who are much worse off than yourself. Replace it with gratitude.
S — Set a goal for yourself. Resolve that if you do have another flare, it will not arise from stress that you could have prevented.

"That's wonderful!" Laura said. "Please send me a copy."

After we hung up, I thought more about the details of each item on the stress list. I wanted to see which ones applied to me and needed my attention.

The following week, Laura telephoned. "Thanks for that acronym. It's great! I wanted to ask you a question.

Would you do something that might help all of us with lupus?"

"Sure, anything," I answered. "Anything at all, you know that. But what can I possibly do to help?"

"Write the story of your experience with lupus and drugs."

"What do you mean?"

"Well, I read your short story that was published and I like the way you write. We need a writer who has lupus and would be willing to do a personal story for a national magazine. There are several that are interested if we can find a writer. We want to make the general public and medical profession more aware of lupus. Also it will help others with the disease. Will you do it?

I was flabbergasted. "Thanks for the compliment, but give me a couple of days to think about it. Sounds like a big undertaking, but an exciting one."

A magazine article on lupus was certainly a project I'd thought about, but my mind formed many questions. I wondered if I could do it justice. Did Laura have a commitment from a magazine? Would I be able to get it published?

Another voice reminded me that it would be a worthwhile undertaking. I wanted to help others just as I had been helped, to pass on the information that had been so freely given me. Perhaps this would be one way I could do it. I called Laura the next day and gratefully accepted. I had already assembled my medical records and a file of notes, but there would be much more to do. More research on the disease itself was the first step, just as I had planned for the book. I reread the pamphlets on lupus. Then would come medical books and interviews with specialists.

I still had trouble saying the name "lupus" to other people. It sounded so menacing. No wonder, as the name was derived from the Latin word meaning *wolf.* In the beginning, the disease was so named because it was thought that the facial rash resembled a wolf bite. Lupus is not contagious, infectious or malignant, yet the name is still repulsive. Maybe it would help if the name were changed. Well . . .

I closed the books and called it a day. What's in a name, anyway? Now who said that! Shakespeare? Go to sleep, Beverly. Enough changing the world for one day!

I tried to keep abreast of all treatments available. The conquering of lupus had become a prime area of medical research in the United States and throughout the world. Scientists were intensely interested in lupus, not only to help those suffering with the disease, but because it could mean finding the key to other closely related disorders, such as rheumatoid arthritis. What better way to get an update than to talk to an expert in the field? I asked Dr. Edmund Dubois, a leading rheumatologist in the field of lupus research and treatment, for an interview. He graciously agreed.

"Dr. Dubois, I appreciate your willingness to give me an update on lupus. For the record, would you first explain what lupus is?"

"Well, there are two forms of lupus erythematosus: discoid LE, the skin form, and systemic LE, the internal form. Neither is contagious. Discoid LE has a specific kind of skin rash with raised, red, scaly areas. Systemic LE is one of the rheumatic diseases. It is a chronic inflammatory disease of the connective tissues affecting many areas of the body in which such tissues are found. Sometimes people have both forms."

"Are we getting any closer today in conquering the disease?" I asked.

"It's hard to say. Theoretically, you're always a day closer, and lupus doesn't have the poor outlook that people used to think it had. About 85 percent of the patients live fifteen to twenty years after you make the diagnosis.

"People have become aware that lupus is not a rare

disease, still there are hundreds of thousands of undiagnosed cases in the United States. But the younger doctors with their training are aware of the disease. There are lupus clinics in nearly every medical school now. Also, with the popular usage of more specific tests like the anit-nuclear antibody test, the disease diagnosis can be confirmed in a lot of equivocal cases."

"Are there still a large number of people who are being treated for other diseases when, in fact, they are victims of lupus?"

"I'm sure there's still a lot of confusion in treatment. Many are being told that they have rheumatoid arthritis; many are being treated for kidney disease that's really lupus. There are atypical skin rashes that are probably lupus that are being called other things. There's still not enough awareness of the disease."

"On the emotional end, " I asked, "like so-called neurotic complaints, is there more awareness now? Or are lupus victims still being treated for neurotic complaints?"

"There are many women in their thirties that feel tired, weak and listless. This can be a manifestation of the disease. Very often they're called neurotic, especially housewives in their thirties."

"What would you suggest to someone who suspects they might have the disease?"

"I think the best thing is to see a rheumatologist, someone who specializes in arthritis and rheumatism. If they have skin lesions, then they should see a dermatologist."

"Considering the importance of a good patient-doctor relationship, how can a person achieve that?"

"I think the doctor has to reassure the patient. By the time most people with lupus get to someone who sees a lot of lupus cases, they are frightened and upset. They think they have a fatal disease that's going to kill them prematurely. They need much reassurance that the disease, in most cases, can be controlled. They need a lot of sympathy."

I thanked Dr. Dubois and expressed my gratitude for all the work he was doing to help in this field.

What a wonderful man, I reflected. With people like him on our side, it's really going to be all right. One day I know they'll find a cure.*

Once I began the manuscript it started to take on proportions I'd never considered. And before I was finished, I had written volumes for this short article. It would be informative, yet it would still just scratch the surface of this subject.

I was delighted when *Woman's World* magazine bought the story. But the most gratifying part occurred after the article was published. The response was overwhelming. Many people with the disease wrote saying that they no longer felt alone. Many others wrote that they now had a better understanding of this mysterious disease. So, a book began to emerge.

Most days I devoted to my work, taking care to pace myself. At night I went to bed, looking forward to morning. When I woke up, I literally bounced out of bed, excited about the new day. I thanked God for that. What a wonder to have fallen asleep without a pill and to have awakened with an eagerness to begin the day.

Each day I meditated, then I could get on with my writing. The day went well as long as I remembered to avoid getting too hungry, too angry, too lonely, or too tired. I had a burning desire to write, to give back some of what I had received. To accomplish this, I knew that I needed time out to take care of myself, to be good to myself. This was not always easy to do, especially as I became more engrossed in my work.

At the end of the day, I continued to thank God for all that He had done for me. For the time, I was no longer overwhelmed by the direction my life had taken after being stricken with an incurable disease. However, before

*Dr. Dubois died February 2, 1985

the year was over, I would learn the true meaning of acceptance, after further pain had invaded my body.

As my disease progressed, I saw noticeable changes in my body. My hair thinned, inflammation invaded my muscles and joints, and my body became stiff and rigid. Most days I couldn't bend to tie my shoelaces, even sitting down. I'd rush through an hour of marketing and errands, everyday living chores, eager to get home and undress again. Even wearing clothes caused discomfort. My fingers wouldn't hold a pen and my concentration waned. My writing came to a standstill. My heart and arteries became involved and my breathing problems increased. Flares came about every six months now. There were illnesses and surgeries, but I found that God never gave me more than I could handle. There was the removal of a tumor. Cancer, I thought. Oh, no. Not that too! I prayed, and I breathed a sigh of relief when the negative results came.

Then in December, heart catheterization was necessary. I needed that diagnostic procedure to ascertain the nature and extent of my heart and artery disease. The catheters are thin, flexible, hollow tubes inserted into the blood vessels and guided through them into the chambers of the heart and mouths of the coronary arteries. Progress of the catheter is monitored by an x-ray TV tube.

I was given a local anaesthetic and they used two different catheters, entering from my right thigh. Blood samples were taken from different areas of the heart, and pressure readings were obtained. During use of the second catheter a contrast dye was used to show the size and shape of the heart chambers and any blocks or narrowings of the arteries. During this catheterization I was on the EKG machine to check my heart action. I didn't have any adverse reactions during the procedure, and I found it fascinating to watch the catheter's movements on the TV screen as the doctor executed the necessary maneuvers.

"This is called angiography," the doctor said. "Heart valve leaks can thus be seen and measured."

I learned the results of the test immediately. My right coronary artery was okay, however the left one had two lesions resulting in a narrowing of 30 and 40 percent. Fortunately, surgery was not necessary. A prior diagnosis of a mitral valve prolapse was verified.

I was told that because of the prolapse, antibiotics should be taken before any dental work, even teeth cleaning, to prevent infection from starting and traveling to the mitral valve area and causing real problems. How I wish I had known of this before I had dental work done in October of that year.

The mitral valve prolapse had been found in 1981, but I had not been warned about taking antibiotics prior to going to the dentist for any work. In the process of preparing a tooth for a crown, the dentist had lacerated an area in my mouth. The result was an infection, a lupus flare, a hospitalization with heart problems, and the need of the catheterization. My pain was consistent with angina, and I obtained relief from nitroglycerin. After my release from the hospital, I wore nitroglycerin patches for many months.

I knew that in the past the three leading causes of death from lupus were kidney failure, infections and central nervous system involvement. Now dialysis was available, as were kidney transplants with new drugs to prevent rejection. Fortunately the disease had not yet attacked my kidneys. However, it was necessary to keep a vigil via tests to watch for that possibility, as lupus kidney involvement is painless. I was also told that infections could complicate lupus and to use special preventive precautions. I needed to avoid people who had infections, give special attention to cleansing open cuts or sores, and report to my doctor any sign of infection. My frequent infections were not only a serious problem in themselves, but they created another problem: the antibiotics killed the good bacteria along with the bad ones! I would then invariably get a secondary infection, also called an opportunistic infection.

With all these infections, I had to take care to get enough of the right drugs to clear the infection, but not enough to become addicted to the drug. I could become spaced out even with antibiotics, so I avoided all pills, even the over-the-counter gems. I hadn't forgotten my Honolulu experiences with those little goodies! I questioned the necessity whenever a pill was prescribed, and I looked the drugs up before using them. Sometimes doctors warned me about medications. For example, when I was put on steroids, it was emphasized that I must not abruptly stop the medication, particularly if it were a large dose of cortisone derivatives. This could lead to a severe lupus flare or even a fatal outcome. Also, pharmacies had sheets of information on most drugs.

Proper rest, nutrition and exercise was the way for me, except in acute situations. I would not be foolish regarding the help medicine could provide, especially in life and death situations. I had no intention of becoming a dead hero, but I would carefully examine my motives before taking any medications. I would use good judgement. Not only mine, but that of my doctor.

Still, my health was deteriorating much too fast for me. I had to be doing something wrong. I knew that I overdid at times. It remained difficult for me to discard old ideas and to pace myself.

9

Putting it all Together

One day, the pain and weakness hit me full force again. My neck and shoulders were spastic. When I telephoned Dr. Darvish, my present rheumatologist, he suggested that I attend an arthritis rehabilitation program. I liked Dr. Darvish from our first meeting and felt I had finally found a competent doctor that I could communicate with, one well informed about lupus. He transmitted positive feelings with his optimism and energy, and he took my complaints seriously. All that, coupled with his warm, cheerful personality was a unique combination. He had genuine concern for his patients. Dr. Darvish and I had a good doctor-patient relationship where we shared in the responsibility of my well-being. He was a rare gem among doctors.

Now I listened as he told me about a rehabilitation program that included lupus patients.

"It's at the Daniel Freeman Hospital in Inglewood," he said. "It's a wonderful program and I think you would benefit from it."

"I've heard of those programs for other diseases, like the one for heart patients, but I didn't know there were any for arthritis or lupus."

"Yes. It's a program for people with arthritis and other rheumatic diseases."

"What happens there?"

"Well, basically, the purpose of the program is to explain to the patient exactly what arthritis is and what we can do in our daily lives to prevent the disease from getting worse, to prevent additional burden to the joints. We have a lot of classes for that number one priority. Number two priority is to promote physical and emotional endurance activities in our daily lives. We stress the emotional as well as the physical because we believe that patients with arthritis have both aspects of pain. By controlling both of them, emotional and physical, we're able to control the arthritis itself. So the program is designed to be preventive as well as curative. We try to teach how to prevent a flare-up, and at the same time try to put the patient into remission."

"What's the difference," I asked, "between this hospital and an acute care section?"

"Here we have a comprehensive program," Dr. Darvish said. "You get psychological support, occupational therapy, and the educational part that patients in acute care are not exposed to. That's the principal difference. We teach that medications are not the sole way to treat arthritis. There are other means.

"Beverly," he continued, "I strongly recommend you try this program. It's a three week commitment, but I know it will help you."

"I'm convinced. Sign me up!"

"I'll have the nurse check to see if a room is available. She'll call you right back—and bring a bathing suit."

"A pool!" I responded. "Great." Things were looking up. A hospital with a swimming pool! I was going to like this. I turned over, smiled to myself and tried to get some rest. Would this shoulder ever stop hurting?

I waited three days, three long, pain-filled days, for an available room. No point in going into the acute care section of the hospital, only to have to be moved. That meant extra blood work, and if nothing else, I would be willing to suffer a lot to avoid that! Besides, I disliked hospitals with a passion and would prefer to wait until there was an opening in the rehabilitation section.

Finally, I was admitted to the hospital's Arthritis and Rheumatic Diseases Rehabilitation Program. Again I felt desperate. The three days had taken their toll. I was sick and tired, weary of having from one to three hospitalizations yearly, each one leaving me physically weaker than before. However, I entered this hospital with an open mind, again willing to go to any lengths to feel better, to get on with living a more normal life.

Even before I was admitted, I knew that this would be a different kind of hospital experience for me. I had been told to bring street clothes, and of course that bathing suit. What fun, I thought. I'm not sure exactly what I expected, but it didn't turn out to be the country club I associated with swimming pools. However, it was in a nice spacious part of the hospital, a bright and cheerful section. Each patient had a large, private room with a giant-size bathroom, set up with helpful aids for those arthritic patients who needed them. The shower-tub even came equipped with a chair. In the beginning, I found all this equipment to be spooky and depressing, but I learned that some of the items made my life easier. When I used them, it took the stress off my joints and preserved my energy. Later, I would attend classes and learn more about joint protection and energy conservation.

The door to my room had a special removable rubber handle which I could easily press down to turn the knob, and the sinks were low enough so that I could even sit down to brush my teeth.

But street clothes or not, large private rooms or not, huge personal bathrooms or not, it was still a hospital. And it brought back memories of another hospital situation I'd been in, the drug rehabilitation one in Honolulu. I wore street clothes there, too. Yes, this place was nice, but it still conjured up too many visions of that horror in my life, making it as vivid as if it were yesterday. A chill ran through my body. I felt misplaced in hospitals, all hospitals, and this one was no exception.

Here at the rehabilitation hospital, in addition to my rheumatologist, were many other arthritis health professionals who would be working with me. Or, as one of the nurses put it, "We'll be working together, you and the staff." Their aim was to help me improve the quality of my life. The professionals and I formed a team, allowing me to be an active participant in the program. My team included my doctor and primary nurse, a physical therapist, an occupational therapist, a clinical social worker, a psychologist, a dietician and a health educator. Their responsibility was to provide me with information, and instruction on how to use the information. My responsibility was to be on time for scheduled activities, to do as much as possible for myself in the daily activities, to communicate my needs, requests and concerns, and to share with my team what I wanted to accomplish.

The rehabilitation program was indeed comprehensive, as Dr. Darvish had told me. It emphasized preparing the patients for an easier life when they left the hospital. The classes included those on arthritis education, diet, exercise, relaxation techniques, and planning and scheduling daily activities, which stressed rest periods.

My prior knowledge was reinforced and expanded upon. It was all put together for me in a program that I would practice in the hospital, so that I could use it on a daily basis at home. Here I would learn about arthritis and lupus, and ways that I could control the disease process. More importantly, I would be using this knowledge every day in the hospital—I would learn by doing.

"Improvement may occur gradually," Dr. Darvish reminded me. "It will require working consistently at your individualized program. And discover all you can about what causes stress for you. Remember that stress and lupus are very closely related. We don't know the cause of lupus, but we do know that stress can play a role in making it worse."

"Doctor, you know I have so many flare-ups, I wonder if I'm ever in remission. Can you pick out one thing, one particular thing, that I and others could learn to control . . ."

"Beverly," he interrupted, "you already know that answer!"

"You mean, pace myself." I laughed. "Slow down?"

"Yes. Pacing is very important. You know when a flare-up is going to happen; you feel it coming up. Instead of pushing yourself, we want you to stop and prevent that flare before it happens. The main thing that you have to learn, Beverly, is what is good for your body and what is bad."

One of the most important and helpful attitudes that the hospital fostered was "wellness" instead of "illness." "Wellness" became a part of our vocabulary. It was stressed throughout the program as being something more than just freedom from symptoms of pain or discomfort.

"Even with a chronic disease you can experience wellness," Dr. Darvish said. He went on to explain that wellness related to the ability of an individual to find personal satisfaction and a sense of purpose in life; that it can be achieved by exploring and examining activities which make you feel good about yourself and your daily routine.

I would learn that an important part of wellness was to create a balance between the energy I expend on work and the revitalization provided by recreation and rest. If work consumed more of my energy than was replenished, my health would suffer. We were encouraged to believe we *could* do many things that well people did, but in our own way, at our own pace.

That was certainly good news! Wellness! What a

great word. "Sure sounds more uplifting than 'sickness,' I told a fellow patient.

"And it's something to strive for," she agreed. I kept this in mind all during my stay at the hospital.

When I entered the hospital program, I could not turn my head, and fatigue had been a major problem for weeks.

"I doubt that I'm physically able to participate in everything," I told the nurse that first night. I wanted to rest, not run around to classes, do exercises and socialize with other people. Also, I knew that my privacy, which I valued highly, was going to be invaded. And I was right. Even in a private room, this program afforded little solitude. But then, hospitals are not noted for privacy. My mind raced and then returned to what the nurse was saying.

"Just do what you can. But you'll be surprised. After a few days, you'll be doing exercises like a pro."

"Well, okay, I'll give it my best shot," I mumbled, feeling disheartened by the word "exercise." I needed rest, not jumping around.

And so my thoughts went that first night. Still, I felt relieved to be there, a place where I knew I would get some help.

Sure enough, exercise was the first activity on the morning agenda. "Meet at the elevator," I was told. "Then we'll go to the pool together." So, at 7 a.m. I put on my bathing suit and my happy face. My body still felt as if it had been hit by a truck, and even the prospect of swimming did not excite me—certainly not at that hour of the day!

Being in water always helped my pain, physically and emotionally, and I had enjoyed swimming long before my illness began. Then after I got sick, I had to temper my water activity to my physical condition, sometimes being able to swim daily, but when in a flare, foregoing swimming for weeks. Then I would have to start slowly again. In the summers I used the pool at home, and in the winters I joined athletic clubs with indoor pools.

"If you swim on a daily basis, you won't have any more back problems," Dr. Darvish had told me when I first met him. This had worked for me.

Now my shoulder and neck hurt and my body was tired. But I wanted to begin this program. I was determined and willing to try anything that would improve the quality of my life. I went to the elevator.

The morning swim never materialized. The pool turned out to be suitable for exercising, but not large enough for swimming. What a disappointment! But I soon realized that it didn't matter—my body couldn't have made it across a pool anyway. Swimming was never allowed during my three-week stay, even when we progressed to a larger pool for endurance exercises. Swimming would come later, at home, when I became stronger.

The physical therapist advised us that stress can cause muscles to become tense and joints to grow stiff, so our exercise plan at the hospital included special range-of-motion exercises twice a day, fifteen minutes for each session. Some of the exercises were done at the pool and some in the exercise room. The exercises would help promote relaxation of the muscles and keep the joints in working order. I was given hints on relaxation for every part of my body and mind. Deep breathing, imagery, and contract-relax were among the kinds of relaxation techniques taught. Endurance-building exercises were recommended for three times a week. These included walking and stationary bicycling, and when I would return home, swimming. We were reminded to do a warm-up before an endurance activity and a stretching cool-down after the activity. Also, we were told to avoid exercise following a meal.

"Always exercise at your own pace," the therapist cautioned. "Learn what that is. Know your limitations. If an exercise causes you pain, don't do it. If you feel dizzy, stop. But don't be lazy either, and do get into a regular routine each day."

For the first few days I couldn't complete most of the exercises, but the rehabilitation team helped me plan a program suited to my individual needs, a self-care schedule that I could follow at home.

"Your fatigue is real," a nurse told me. "You can't see it, but you know that it exists. It's one of the hidden features of lupus, and this program will help you deal with it. It will take time and perseverance on your part, but it will be worth it. You will be controlling your body and your life, and that will make you feel better."

I learned how to plan my activities according to my available energy, to be attentive to my body's signals and not fight the fatigue, to accept my limitations, and the importance of exercise.

In one of our first classes, they talked about normal, healthy joints and what happens to them in the rheumatic diseases. In another class, we were instructed in how to best use our body to help control the joint changes caused by arthritis. I discovered ways to lift, hold, and move objects to protect my joints.

"Use the stronger joints whenever possible," the instructor said. "For example, use the shoulder rather than the elbow, the elbow rather than the wrist, the wrist rather than the fingers."

I was taught to sit whenever possible, not stand, to lie down rather than sit, and to slide objects instead of lifting them.

"Lead upstairs with your strong foot and lead

downstairs with your weak one," Pat said. "And when you're writing, don't forget to stretch your fingers every ten minutes."

Proper body mechanics for everyday living were suggested, ranging from how to make the bed to dressing myself, from driving a car to working at my computer. Every day we were instructed in new ways to conserve energy. Everything was geared to helping us become more independent.

I used many aids which I later bought to utilize at home, including special scissors, a giant-size cutting knife, lever knobs for my doors, an elevated toilet seat, a jar opener, key ring, coffee cup, sponge pen and pencil holders, all designed to minimize the stress on my joints. At home, the stiffness in my fingers had hampered the use of scissors. Now, with the hospital's unique scissors, it presented no problem.

Each day I heard things like "pace yourself" and "learn your limitations."

In the classes on diet, the nutritionist advised us to read the labels on food items, to avoid salt, sugar and other food additives, limit intake of soft drinks to less than five per week, avoid large doses of vitamins, specific foods or herbal remedies, and heed various other nutritional policies, some of which I already had incorporated in my life.

We spent one morning each week in a special kitchen where we were taught easy methods of preparing meals, another lesson in joint protection. Amazing cooking aids were demonstrated, and those, too, I purchased for use at home. Anything that would make my life easier and less painful; that's what it was all about.

But the greatest part of the program was not what I learned. The exceptional thing about this approach was that with the help of an outstanding staff, I lived it. For three weeks, I had qualified, compassionate staff members pushing me and helping to do the things they competently taught. Each day, I followed a routine using the information, aids and suggestions provided, a routine that I could take home with me. This was a practical, comprehensive method of instructing me on how to live with lupus and arthritis.

At the formal classes I studied ways to control the disease process, but much of what I learned came about by informal means, in daily therapy, in talking to patients and staff members, in the use of suggested aids.

I began to really see the benefits of adequate rest for emotional fitness as well as physical fitness. It was an essential and helpful coping tool.

Along with the others in the group, I was encouraged to talk about my progress on a daily basis, to recognize both the good and the bad days. And once a week we had a team meeting to discuss areas of improvement and areas needing more work.

During my hospital stay, I experienced a variety of emotions, vacillating mostly among anxiety, anger and rage, and then, ultimately, exhilaration. This was not unusual. I had been told that some negative emotions might surface, as well as the joy at the improvement I would make.

"Those are all natural responses," I read in the manual provided for patients. "Learning to cope with these feelings is the first step to wellness. You are not alone."

As it turned out, all of these things were discussed at meetings with other patients. When the feelings became too painful, I considered talking to the psychologist, especially since stress also continued to be a major concern in my well-being. I didn't know how to become aware of the early signs of tension and stress, so I could stop when those signs appeared. If I dealt with stressful situations, rather than ignoring them, maybe I could prevent them from happening again. How should I handle this? Should I go to the therapist? I repeatedly asked myself that question. In Honolulu, my experiences with a therapist had been disastrous, leading me deeper into drug addiction. Would it be different now? I wondered. Well, a psychologist's services were available to me here, so why not give it a try. At least talk to him, I told myself. I certainly could use some suggestions on this stress item. I made an appointment for the following day.

"Everybody is subject to stress," said Dr. Tim Field, the senior medical psychologist at the hospital. "There are three main components of stress reduction. It isn't just a matter of watching your diet and exercising, although those are two important aspects. There's also a third aspect, and that is mental health. This psychological factor is the one most people neglect and then wonder why they don't feel good, even though they exercise and watch their diet every day. We forget to include the psychological aspect in terms of stress reduction."

"How does this relate to illness?" I asked.

"The major relationship is that stress causes dramatic changes in the physical functions of the body just as illness does. Any illness automatically drains the body, so when you add stress, that drains you even further and can make the illness much worse than it needs to be.

"Or stress can set you up to develop an illness. While it doesn't specifically cause illnesses, such as cancer or arthritis or lupus, it reduces the body's ability to fight the illness off. So what you have is a situation of a system in our body that's weak. Add stress to that system, and the body might not be able to defend itself against the illness as it normally would. It can't fight both the illness and the stress."

"Going back to lupus, do you think that stress is the single-most prevalent cause of a flare-up?"

"I wouldn't say 'single-most,' but I'd say it's definitely one of the top causes of flare-ups. When we see how stress affects the body physically, it's understandable how emotional tension can lead to a flare-up. However, most people don't understand this."

"I understand how stress can cause a flare-up. I've seen it happen with me. Now, if I learn how to cope with stress and to eliminate distress from my life, can I prevent flare-ups?"

"You can't always totally prevent them, but you can dramatically reduce the incidence of them. That's true with any illness. People who take care of themselves have fewer colds, flu symptoms and can fight off all illnesses better. When stress is allowed to build up, it weakens the body's immune system.

"With lupus, the body's immune system is already weakened and works against itself, so stress reduction is even more important."

"How about some good methods of doing this? I've simplified my life as much as possible and have learned ways of coping with stress, but it still sends me into a flare. Any suggestions on stress reduction?"

"It requires a lot of things. Number one, the basic physical facts of diet and exercise are important, as we mentioned before—physical stresses on the body can have a profound effect. Then there's relaxation to calm down the machinery of the mind.

"We basically have two sides to our brain, and each has its own function. The left side is our logical, very analytical side, our language side. This side causes much of our stress, because it's the side that's saying, 'You should be doing this; you should be doing that. You've got to push yourself harder.' It's that part of our brain that never shuts up and its chatter can keep you from sleeping.

"Relaxation techniques stop that left, chatty side of the brain from taking over, allowing the right, creative side to balance it out. They tap into that creative process, the relaxed part of our mind, and wipe out much of the stress."

"So, stress can tear anyone's body down," I said. "But there is something we can do about the stress in our lives."

"Yes," he agreed. "Even if you've been under stress for thirty or more years, and even if your health problems seem so serious you think nothing will help, it's no reason not to try stress reduction. It's not hopeless and it will always make a difference. You're never too young or too old to learn relaxation techniques and to apply them."

"Yes, I remember another doctor telling me the same thing," I said. "So I have to learn how to better clear out my mind, to open it up and relax, perhaps using tapes or readings or some other meditation process. When I relax my mind, the body follows. I have to find whatever means works best for me, so I guess if a method gives me a good day, then I must be on the right track."

"Exactly," Dr. Field concurred. "Relaxation can also extend your life because of the biological effect stress has. It actually produces chemical changes in the brain."

"That's interesting," I said.

Just then a nurse entered the room to remind Dr. Field that he was scheduled to lead a class on relaxation techniques in five minutes.

"Oh, that's one class I don't want to miss!" I said. "Thanks for talking with me. Afterwards, I'm going to make a list of the stressful conditions in my life, and try to find a way to avoid or relieve each of those situations."

I had entered the rehabilitation hospital feeling depressed and in incredible pain, barely able to move. Now, three weeks later, I was walking out, pain-free and in good spirits. Best of all, I had been given coping and controlling tools to use at home in my daily life. The benefits of rehabilitation so impressed me that I excitedly told all my friends about the program. One day I called Parks to discuss the points that had been stressed at the hospital. They were:

1. Develop a positive attitude.
2. Adhere to a well-balanced diet.
3. Be sensitive to your environment.
4. Reduce daily stress situations.
5. Meet all of your health care needs.
6. Understand and express your feelings.
7. Follow a daily exercise program.
8. Protect your joints.
9. Get adequate rest and relaxation.
10. Recognize your progress—Be good to yourself.

"Maybe we should do an acronym on that!" he said. We both laughed and decided to save that task for another day. Besides, I was anxious to get to a rap group that was meeting that afternoon.

10
Second Self-help Session

When I arrived at the meeting, Mary, a thin attractive woman in her forties, began to share.

"One of the worst complications of my lupus is an esophagus problem. My throat has to be dilated every three or four months, otherwise I start choking on food. Also, I have central nervous system involvement with hallucinations. At one time I was completely out of my mind, couldn't answer the phone; I wasn't even rational enough to doubt my own sanity. I wasn't aware of lupus or anything else, though; I was happy."

"Guess that was a protective mechanism, or something, that your head did!"

"How long ago was that?"

"Well," Mary continued, "I was diagnosed in '78 when I had a flare. I had only been married for two years. I'm not married now—lupus broke up my marriage. I'm lucky that my ex-husband is still a good friend, though. He takes me grocery shopping and to the doctors.

"Before the lupus flare, I had a job that I had wanted all my life, as an escrow secretary, and I'd just been promoted to escrow officer. One day I got a severe sunburn in my back yard. In addition, I was very worried about not being able to do exchanges of real estate at work and had become obsessed with the thought. I think the stress of that plus the sunburn caused the flare, and I ended up for the first time completely out of my mind, completely paralyzed. I couldn't even turn over. I was in the hospital for two months that time, and since then, I've had many one-month stays in hospitals. The shortest time was two weeks.

"I was in the child-bearing years when lupus first started. I had ulcers on every finger and they oozed, and I also had severe pain in my joints. But, prior to 1978, no doctor could diagnose what was wrong. My circulation was bad and I had to wear gloves, especially at night. I have Raynaud's disease, too. I suspected lupus because I had read about it in a book. I asked the doctor to do tests for this, but they apparently came out negative. He couldn't help me. When I changed doctors, the new doctor diagnosed it.

"I've had kidney involvement and was completely bedridden for several years and confined to a wheelchair for many years after that. I couldn't write at all, and I had to sign a power of attorney over to my husband in order to cash my disability checks. I couldn't even sign anything. An 'x' was the best I could manage.

"I remember that during one of my attacks, I couldn't read because my eyesight was going. I began hallucinating. Later, when they showed me some writing I had done, I was shocked to see that it was just a bunch of scrawls."

"You've really made tremendous progress," Terry said, and we all nodded in agreement.

"That's true. And thank God for my second husband. He took me to every lupus meeting and, even though we're not married anymore, he is still involved in taking care of me. I had three boys in my first marriage, and I'm grateful that I had them when I did. I had the bad flare when they were teenagers, and afterwards I couldn't take care of them and myself too. He was a better father than their real dad.

"I finally got out of the wheelchair. I learned to walk and to write, started going out of the house more and became more functional. But recently I've had severe depression. The doctor gave me something for insomnia and even though I had a bad experience with the medication, I have to take it because I have a sleep disorder caused by lupus."

"That's part of the lupus? Insomnia?"

"Yes. He called it a sleep disorder, and I guess it occurs frequently. I'm down to thirteen prescriptions now because I'm in remission. He's starting to take me off medications because last month I got a severe reaction to one of the pills. A rash. I couldn't believe that. It wasn't like I was taking a *new* pill that my body wasn't used to, but I guess my body just got fed up with that pill. So he took me off it and the rash went away, gradually. I was up to 120 mil. of cortisone in the hospital, and I ballooned to 170 pounds!

"Emotionally, I'm happy when I can come off my medication. I feel that I've really done something!"

"You really have," Terry said. "You feel good because you can decrease those dosages, but I also know what's going to happen, in my case, with a decrease in dosage. I'll start to feel renewed symptoms."

"You anticipate these?"

"Yes. I know they're coming."

"Don't you think that perhaps worrying and anticipating the symptoms might have something to do with them occurring?"

"Yes, that's true, to some extent. There's a feeling of accomplishment knowing that I'm decreasing the meds, but also anxiety."

"What you are saying, Dianne, is that maybe if you anticipate that you're going to feel all right, perhaps you will?"

"Maybe," Dianne said. "But I don't want to put it

that simplistically. I think that perhaps your antenna is out there looking for all the bad feelings. When I'm coming down off pills, it's scary because I know I won't feel good and I know it's going to take me weeks before I feel better. Also, if I'm off drugs and I get sick and have to go back on them, the drug works slowly, and I know that it will be a long haul before I feel any relief."

"Why do they take you off medication if you feel so good on it?"

"Because of the long-term side effects, the doctors are concerned about high dosages."

"It's sort of a double-edged sword."

"Getting back to what Mary was saying about not being diagnosed, it was years before I found out what was wrong with me. I went to a dentist, who later told me that he thought I had lupus. Imagine, a dentist! But nobody could diagnose me until I went to a place here. The doctor who diagnosed me saved my life, although he didn't think I would make it. I had pericarditis."

"That's inflammation of the lining in the heart. It's pretty common with lupus patients. What were your symptoms?"

"Pain in the heart—so I knew something was wrong, but I didn't know what. Imagine, a dentist!"

"When you mentioned a dentist," I began, "it reminded me of the florescent lights they use. Dianne and I were discussing florescent lighting the other day, and I'd like to talk more about it."

"Everybody knows me on that subject!" Dianne laughed. "If they know me they know about lighting."

"I'm very sensitive to certain lighting," Wally said.

"Really?" I said. "I am, too. I would get ill, but it was a long time before I related it to lighting. Sometimes, I would go to the dentist and get ill from the light he uses."

"And I don't," Mary said. "Bev, we've been in the

same room and you get ill from the lighting, but it doesn't bother me."

"Are you not sensitive to the sun, Mary?"

"Oh, yes! I'm very sensitive. I can't go out to dump the trash without using a sun screen—my nose will turn completely red."

"Yet, fluorescent lights don't bother you."

"Right."

"Everyone's lupus is their personal lupus, as we said before. No two are alike."

"Crazy, isn't it. That's why it's so difficult to diagnose."

"Personally, after reading so much about photosensitivity, I would never push it too much. My dermatologist tells *all* of his patients to use sun protection, to stay out of the sun. And in this day and age we know that the sun can cause skin cancer and that it speeds up the aging process. They're now saying that we're going to have even more cancers because of the ozone layer being depleted."

"My eyes are very sensitive to sunlight."

"I wear dark protective lenses. Medicare doesn't cover it, but I have cataracts from the medications and I have prescription glasses."

"You can have your lenses treated for ultra violet radiation protection," I said. "It's very reasonable. I just had it done to my glasses and it cost fourteen dollars."

"I had it done, too, because I'm so photosensitive," Dianne said. "It doesn't make sense to take chances when ultraviolet blocking is so reasonable. And the suncreens are also great."

"Yes, the chemical sunscreens are wonderful."

"What do you mean by chemical sunscreens—as opposed to what other?"

"Well, there's physically shading yourself, such as using a wide-brim hat and long sleeves. I wear long sleeves outside and then use a chemical on my skin that provides a sunscreen."

"Okay, I understand."

"It used to be that the only protection a lupus patient had against the sun was zinc oxide, and to wear a big floppy hat. But there's reflection from your surroundings when you wear a hat, so you don't get enough protection. Now we have lots of chemical sunscreens available that are very protective."

"You have to read what you're buying, though. Some of them are worthless."

"My friend's dermatologist told him that he was allergic to the perfume in most sunscreens: it turned his skin red in just a few days."

"Wally, when did your disease start?" Dianne asked.

"It was a couple years ago," Wally said. "I flew fighter planes in the Marine Corps. One time, four years ago, I failed a flight physical for an unknown reason. It's not too much different than sending paperwork off for an insurance policy. They take the results of your tests—bloodwork, x-rays, EKG's, and so on—and send them off to headquarters, who sends you back a piece of paper saying that you're good for another year. Mine came back with red marks all over it, so from that point on I wasn't allowed to fly until they investigated the problem.

"My diagnosis was anemia, but when they investigated it further, they kept coming up blank. I was stationed in the southern part of Arizona, at that time—a great place to have lupus! You know, where the sun always shines! Of course, I was a member of perhaps the healthiest group of men in the United States. There are no sick people there, so nothing could be wrong with me, right? I thought I'd just take some iron pills, and I'd be over it and everything would be okay. I was also doing a lot of fishing, in

March and April when the sun shines intensely in Arizona. I began developing these sunburns that wouldn't go away. Then, slowly but surely, I started having total engulfment of discoid type lupus all over my body, but, at that time, I had no idea what it was. There's no military medical facility there, except the dispensary, so I saw the only dermatologist in town. He said, 'I think you have something called lupus, but as best as I can tell, since you don't exhibit anything else, you may just have what's known as discoid lupus. It's going to present a lot of problems for you.' And then he described some of them to me.

"They terminated my flight status but let me remain in the military. Then, about four months later, I started developing some severe problems and couldn't walk. Then, I couldn't even get up out of a chair, and I was referred to the military here in California and put under the care of a dermatologist. He gave me a medication that cleared my skin problem, but my joint pains became more severe. I asked about seeing another doctor, because I didn't think the treatment was helping overall. The doctor said, 'Hey, you're going to be all right. You have what is known as sub-acute cutaneous lupus. You're not having any other problems.' They sent me back to Arizona, and I returned about once a month to California for tests because of possible medication side effects. All this time, I was failing, and finally one weekend, my temperature went up to 106 degrees and I couldn't get out of bed at all. I could hardly breathe . . ."

"This is not sub-acute!"

The laughter was contagious, and we all participated in the much needed release.

"All this time," Wally continued, "I'm thinking that surely these doctors wouldn't be wrong—they know what they're doing. That's probably why I don't have much faith in dermatologists now."

"There are a lot of knowledgeable ones, though."

"I know. I just had that bad experience. Finally they flew my wife and me from Arizona to California. I was immediately admitted to the hospital and told that I had all kinds of problems stemming from systemic lupus.

"I was in the hospital for a couple months with many ups and downs. A lot of drugs were necessary because of the kidney disease from the lupus, and I also had lung disease."

"How did you feel having to go through all this after being told that it was minor?"

"I wasn't quite sure that I was going to make it, and psychologically I was very upset. I also had a lot of denial and that eventually caused many problems. I wouldn't face what I had. I was released from the hospital, and within a month I almost had myself convinced that I had been in the hospital for an infection. Now they had it cured and I was all right, so I went back to work in Arizona, not flying but doing all the office jobs. I was working about fourteen hours a day, immersing myself in my job, but I was also on steroids. Then they slowly started tapering me off them, and I was back to doing all the things I normally did, thinking that everything was okay.

"In the meantime, my wife was saying, 'Hey, you better take it easy." I didn't listen to her any more than I listened to my rheumatologist in California. I was going my own way, doing what I thought was right. About four months later, I was flown back to California again, back in the same place only this time physically worse than before. I was in intensive care for about two weeks. The doctors came in to tell me that there came a time in everybody's life when you have to face facts. 'We've done everything we can for you, and we don't know at this point whether you'll make it or not.' So everyone was prepared for my dying, but I disappointed them all. I lived through it, and I finally realized that I had something that, sooner or later, I'd have to deal with and I could no longer keep looking the other way. The 'later' had come. I was very fortunate because my wife was probably much better versed on what was wrong with me than many spouses. She knew more of what was going on and the things I needed to do, than I did. She was very, very good, and if it hadn't been for her, I don't think that I would have made it through everything."

"How lucky you are that you have her."

"I know. Also, I went to lupus meetings and rap sessions in Arizona. I was the only male, but that didn't matter. I listened to the problems that these people had and started to realize I was in a bad situation and had to contend with it. But I'm fortunate, maybe more fortunate than most people with lupus, because I was retired with a pension from the military. Although I'm not wealthy, I don't have financial problems that can come with not being able to work. Plus, I have very strong emotional support from my wife. Something made me realize that I needed to consider the whole picture as far as what life had dealt me. I got a bad deal with lupus, but still, as I said, I'm very, very fortunate, more so than a lot of people.

"I had a life that was a lot of fun; there isn't anything I would rather have done. I can't do it anymore, but I was lucky that I got to do it as long as I did."

"In a way, it's like your other self dying, isn't it?" Dianne said. "That self is gone, so you have a new self."

"Right. I'm a completely different person. That's a good way to put it."

"I guess the problem I had most difficulty dealing

with was self-image," Terry interjected. "I went from 170 to 240 pounds in just six weeks. I've got stretch marks that a pregnant woman would be proud of!"

"Weren't you angry?"

"Oh, I was angry. I was scared. And I didn't want any of my friends to see me. I have to admit that, even now, although I've lost most of the weight, I still have those fears. I'm embarrassed. It's hard to explain. I know that these things are present, these feelings, and I know that I shouldn't feel that way, and that my physical problems are nothing to be ashamed of. But, it really doesn't make it any better. The feelings are still there."

"You mean on a logical level you know this," Dianne said, "but on another level, it hurts."

"Exactly. And I know that even though my friends understand to a point . . . I still don't feel good about myself, and that almost surely is communicated to them."

"You mention friends," Dianne said. "One thing I've learned is that there are friends and there are acquaintances. And boy, you sure learn which ones are acquaintances! Fast!"

"That's exactly right," we all chimed together.

"And I've lost no friends," Dianne continued.

"I sure have!" Terry said.

"Then I would say those people weren't really friends. They were acquaintances."

"Was it because you couldn't do what you used to do for them or with them?"

"I don't know," Terry said. "Two of my friends got kinda mad. I think because they were working and I couldn't always hold a job. When they came to visit me in the hospital, they seemed to feel uncomfortable. They don't want to handle it."

"They can't handle it," Dianne explained.

"I guess that's true. Emotionally they just can't

handle it."

"I think it's the same thing you once talked about," Wally said. "Like being in a wheelchair or walker when someone comes up and will speak to the person that's with you, rather than to you. That's their discomfort with the situation. People are almost afraid of someone who has a disability. They will almost act like you're not there or, in our case since we look okay, like we're not sick."

"They deny that you're sick. Maybe they're afraid to identify with you."

"Not that they don't want to, they just can't understand," Wally continued. "For example, how can I understand death when I'm a kid. I go to see my grandpa and someone tries to explain that he's dead because of a disease. All I know is that I miss him, so I cry because he's gone. I wouldn't have been able to understand someone with cancer if I hadn't gotten lupus. I couldn't relate to all these things, to a chronic illness.

"And being young, we're forced into these emotions before we've learned to understand the concept of mortality. Most people aren't forced to realize their own mortality until they're much older."

"Yes, that's what I meant earlier," Terry said. "All that I've gone through in the past couple years, most people don't experience in a lifetime."

"But then maybe you're not so bad off for the experience."

"No, I'm not. I feel like I'm going to be a happier person and enjoy what's left. And I'm going to enjoy that a lot more than probably my dad would. Well, it's like I lost my health, but then I got some of it back and I know what I lost. I can laugh it off because I know what I've got and I see things as they really are.

"In some ways I feel lucky to have gotten lupus and survived it and grown through the experience."

"What else can they do to you?" Terry said.

We all laughed.

"No joke. Honestly, when you think about it . . ."

"Well, they can do a lot," Dianne said. "I have a real mild case. I haven't had the life-threatening situations, but I still have been able to appreciate having the disease and dealing with the mortality."

"This may be a little naive on my part, but I honestly believe now that there isn't anything that could happen to me that I couldn't handle. I really believe that. I don't know where that comes from."

"An inner feeling . . ."

"Right. I don't know where it comes from. Maybe it comes from someone else, maybe the men's group I've been going to. I get a lot out of that group. Maybe it's being around other people and hearing their stories. Maybe it comes from my wife. I don't know, but I honestly believe what I was saying."

"Don't downplay yourself. You can hear everything, but you still have to make sense of it."

"I think you'll eventually come to more inner strength," Dianne said to Terry.

"Right. A few months ago, I had some flash-backs to the emotions. I find that prayer helps a lot. I thought I was a tough person, but I found out that I'm not."

"I think everyone in this room is a survivor. We've survived against tremendous odds. And what you were saying before is that there are no big deals left anymore."

"No shocks," Wally said, and then spoke to Claire, the retired nurse in our group. "One time, you said that you felt sorry for the young people. I feel the other way. I'm speaking as one of those young people. I mean, you've spent your entire life working and pursuing your goal, and now when you could relax and enjoy the remaining years, that's taken away. Now we could go round and round as to which one's worse, but I think they're equally bad."

"Well, I'm glad I don't see it that way," Claire laughed. "I'm like Terry. I have a very profound faith that has helped me through, and if I should just fall asleep for good tonight, then fine, my life has been good. Our lives are totally in the hands of God."

"Spirituality is something you can't really get by just reading books. You have to feel it inside."

"Right, and I do. I've done a lot of growing in that area, and I like the serenity I feel now."

"I miss the hard and fast life I had in the military," Wally said.

"Would you want to go back to that life?"

"Yes, ma'am. It's in my blood. I would never have given up flying until the day. . . "

"Well, flying, yes. But that doesn't necessarily go with a hard and fast life."

"Well . . ." We all laughed.

"Please don't misunderstand," Wally explained. "I don't mean in the morality sense. I mean the intensity with which one pursues a career."

"You can progress in your faith in the same way, and that can be satisfaction and gratification in itself."

"Well, yes, but this might be where I differ from you and others. I'm not a profoundly religious person. However, I do have spiritual pursuits in my life. I work with deaf people in rehabilitation, and I get my spiritual gratification from that sort of activity. I have to do what works for me."

"Yes, and I share some of the feelings you get from that kind of work. The last five years of my career was as a school nurse for 125 orthopedically handicapped children. That was the most rewarding time of my entire working career.

"They had something special, and I learned many lessons from them regarding the deeper meaning of life."

"Like I said before," Dianne interjected, "I'm lucky with my understanding family, but, like Wally, I would go back to my other life in a minute. I really would. I had a very active life, physically. Very sportsminded. I took care of the yard and did the painting. But my life now is also satisfying, in a way that I didn't have before. I do stop and smell the roses now, not just the manure I'm planting them with. That's the key difference. I would never have done that five years ago."

"Mary, you've talked about the difficulties of living alone."

"Yes, Mary, I remember that," I said. "Actually, I only know a few people with lupus who live alone. Either they're married or living with family or friends. Mary and I are the only ones here today who aren't married. I think there are special problems involved when you live alone, just as you have special ones when you're living with others. You were saying that's part of why you're feeling so depressed."

"Bev, that's true," Mary responded. "It's because I don't have anyone around to emotionally support me. My kids are all grown and living away from me. I miss just having someone to hold me and hug me. It's lonely."

"I think," Terry began, "when I was separated from my wife for that short time, a month or maybe it was a week . . ."

"Twenty minutes maybe!" Dianne interrupted.

"Whatever." Terry laughed. "That time was scary. When I was feeling good, I could cope with living by myself. But I never felt as lonely as when I found out that I had lupus and I didn't have anybody there. My dad came down to visit me for a week, and that was nice, but it was hard on him. I was almost in a coma at that time. I kept thinking that I'd better get up and move around or I was never going to wake up. Then I went into the hospital. I was so pale that the staff was freaking out, and I asked the doctor if they had checked my blood sugar. 'No,' he answered, 'but I bet you know better than we as to what to do.' And I did—I'd been in the hospital so many times. So, three days later they took my blood sugar."

"Don't you think that parents have a hard time dealing with it when children get sick?"

"My dad had kidney problems when he was younger, and his dad had a rough time handling that."

"It's very hard for parents to deal with lupus or any other disease. 'My child can't have it. If I ignore it, it's going to go away.' That makes it harder for the child, no matter what age. Also, there's the denial that goes on with all the family, not only parents."

"My dad and my wife were the worst. My mom keeps me going, but Dad doesn't want to hear about it."

"Some parents may feel guilty, thinking that maybe they transmitted this disease to the child."

"Yes, and then sometimes there's a lot of worrying about whose side of the family it's on. 'It's got to be on your side because my side has perfect genes,' and so on!

"Let me relate a story that illustrates this," Diane continued. "I talked to one lady for over a year about her 14-year-old grandson who was ill with lupus. It was always in a gruff vice that she would say, 'it's my daughter-in-law who has lupus. She's the one who passed it on to the boy. My poor grandson is in this condition because of my daughter-in-law.' Not too long ago I heard again from this lady. Her daughter had been diagnosed with lupus, and she personally was being tested for the possibility. Some of the aches and pains that she'd had over the years most likely had been lupus all this time, as opposed to just aches and pains. So, her grandson may have gotten it not only from the daughter-in-law, but from the grandmother too! The thing about this sad, ironic story is that no one is sure where the boy got it."

"Lupus is not just any one thing. There has to be more than one factor involved. It may be that a person is predisposed to it genetically, but that doesn't mean you're going to get it. It has to be triggered."

"Stress has a lot to do with it. You can have stress at work, maybe feeling you're not qualified for this or that. I went through a lot mentally before I got ill. I had to move—they sold the house we were renting. So, with two kids, I had to find another place. Within that month, I got clobbered. My kidneys shut down and freaked the doctor, totally surprised him."

"Okay, that was a trigger, but you wouldn't have had that happen unless you were predisposed to it in the first place."

"Right. Stress doesn't cause the disease."

"Maybe not, but it almost killed me!"

"It can definitely kill you. They're talking about women and breast cancer, and they're saying that the autoimmune system has a lot to do with controlling cancer, that women are getting cancer because of stress in their lives."

"These are all situations where the people are predisposed to having that disease."

"And there's more to breast cancer than stress. They're blaming fat, high fat, and nutritional problems, and studying whether it's inherited. It's more than just stress."

"Your body can only handle so much. If it's trying to fight off stress, it can't also fight a disease that you're predisposed to."

"Bev, didn't you just talk to someone about this? As some of you know, Beverly was in an arthritis rehabilitation program. Why don't we take a coffee and stretch break and you can tell us all about it. I know you've been bursting to do that!"

I laughed. "I really have. It's exciting to know that this kind of treatment is available for people with lupus and other rheumatic diseases. It sure helped me, and I saw many other miracles as a result of this program."

During the break, I shared my three-week hospital experience. Then we went on with the discussion.

"I think that most all my flares begin with over-extending myself or because of some kind of prolonged stress. I still go through that bit of, 'Well, what's the worst that can happen if I keep pushing myself?' What happens is that I get ill! I suffer for the dumb things that I do. Other people may not understand when I have to pace myself, but I think most of it is me."

"You mean, you make too many demands of yourself?"

"Yes."

"I have that problem too. All I can say is that it's gotten better over the years."

"Some of that maybe goes back to saying 'no' without feeling guilty."

"That's it exactly!"

"It's like learning to sit down *before* you get tired. It's the same principle."

"It's like giving your body permission to rest; that's the same as giving yourself permission to say 'no.' "

"The people I know don't understand the disease, and they don't seem really interested in it. I don't want anyone to feel sorry for me—I just want them to understand."

"Right!"

"This may be the only place you'll get that understanding, here and other places like this."

"It's hard to explain lupus to someone. Too many

have never even heard of it. I think the best spokesperson for lupus was Victoria Principal. Here was someone really recognizable and really attractive, talking of her fear that she might get lupus because her mother has it. That really got people's attention."

"When somebody well-known gets a chronic illness, it really spreads an awareness of the disease. Look what Rock Hudson did to further the awareness of AIDS and get people interested in research. I don't mean that I would want anyone to get lupus. I feel sad when I hear that animals are being used and infected with the disease for research. It breaks my heart that they give these poor little macaque monkeys lupus by feeding them alfalfa seeds."

"Feeding them what?"

"Alfalfa seeds."

"Really? That's my favorite food!"

"You might get better if you stop eating it!"

"What if you felt great just by not eating alfalfa sprouts?"

"Okay! Enough! No more alfalfa!"

"Not to change the subject," Dianne began, "but one thing we haven't really talked about is the loneliness and isolation that can come with this disease."

"I felt a lot of that when I was first diagnosed," I said. "And at times, I still do, though not as much. In the beginning I thought that I was the only person in the world who had this problem, this horrible-sounding disease."

"Yes, I felt that way," Dianne said, while all of us nodded our heads in agreement. "I looked in the phone book and couldn't find any lupus groups here—at that time there weren't any. So that made it worse. I thought it must be a very rare disease—everything else has a foundation or society, and I had never talked to anyone who had the disease.

I had never even heard of it. I thought I was some kind of weirdo with this strange disease. When I told my neighbor I'd been diagnosed with something called lupus, she said, 'Well, leave it to you to get something different.' She had never heard of it either. I felt totally isolated. I tried to explain to her, but I didn't really understand it myself, so I couldn't explain it to anyone else."

"I remember the day my doctor told me, 'Oh your test came out positive on this one thing.' I thought, positive, oh that's good, I'm all for positive. 'You have systemic lupus.' What the heck is that, I asked him, and he went into his office to get the number of a lupus group. 'I'm not going to explain it to you. I want you to go see these people. Here's the phone number.' And I called."

"You won't hear that very often. There are a few doctors in town that will send you to us, but not many."

"That is unusual."

"Very unusual. You were lucky."

"Right. And then he says, 'Well, I know you're in a bind and that your insurance only covers 80 percent. I won't take any more from you!' That guy has been really great, beside the fact that he saved my life!"

"Getting back to loneliness," Mary interrupted, "don't you think that has something to do with being single?"

"Oh, no. It's an internal thing."

"Yes, but being alone and being responsible for yourself . . ."

"No, not that. That's a separate problem from the loneliness that you're feeling. It doesn't matter whether you're with somebody or not."

"What I meant is," Mary continued, "it helps to be with someone who understands and can give you a hug once in a while, not to be alone. If something happens to me . . . like you were saying, when you were separated from your wife."

"When I have the vibes of someone else in the apartment, I don't get these awful lonely feelings. Sometimes at night my faith flies out the window and I feel very alone, like I'm going to die. And I don't want to die alone. I don't know where these fears are coming from, but if there's someone sleeping in the next room, or if I'm visiting my family and not alone at night, I may have the same physical pain, but just the vibes of someone else there helps me not to feel that fear."

"That's exactly what happens with me. I really understand what you're saying, but I don't know the answer."

"My wife and I sleep in our large bed with her hanging onto one side and me hanging onto the other because our body temperatures are different. Still, I know she's there."

"Pets can do that for people, don't you think? I mean squelch the loneliness; just having something alive in the house helps."

"Yes, I guess so. I have a dog and that is comforting."

"No pets are allowed in my apartment building, so I bought a stuffed animal. I feel like a kid snuggling with my little dog at night. We watch TV together and—okay, so I'm weird!"

We all giggled and Mary said, "I don't think you're weird. Whatever works. However, dogs, stuffed or real, can't drive! I can't get around easily, and my ex-husband takes me to the market, to doctors, and does a lot of things for me that I'm unable to do. A lot of my depression is due to the fact that he's now dating someone and is more involved with her than with me. They might get married.

"You see, I was so brain-involved in the beginning

with this disease that even though I was really in love with him, I asked him to move out. My head just wasn't working right. I was going through bad seizures. I'm still in love with him, but he says he doesn't love me anymore. Still, he's very supportive and helpful, maybe because he's been disabled himself in the past and knows what it's like."

"Mary, how did you know you had CNS involvement?"

"My doctors told me. Through tests, I guess. I was completely out of it. When I was first hospitalized, the doctor used to come into the room everyday and quiz me. 'What does it mean when you say that people who live in glass houses shouldn't throw stones?' he would ask, or 'How much is 100 minus seven?' "

"Whatever happened to 'what's two and two?' "

"Ask me that other one, seven from 100, ask me that one at 7:30 in the morning—I don't think I'd know the answer!"

Mary laughed along with the group and continued with her story.

"A lot of my memory is gone. Sometimes certain memories come into my mind, but some years are totally gone."

"Were those the first symptoms?"

"No. I went to the doctor for severe joint pains years before my memory loss."

"The reason I'm asking is that my doctor told me that if I didn't have CNS in the beginning, it wasn't likely to occur now, which is encouraging."

"Generally speaking, it's been documented that what's going to happen to you with lupus is going to happen within the first couple years. So if you're going to have kidney problems, for example, you'll probably have them in the first couple years, same as with the other organs. No hard and fast rules, but generally speaking, statistically speaking, I'm going to remain with the same problems because I've had lupus for so many years. There might be some changes, but no big surprises down the line, no major episodes. My doctors are not expecting kidney or heart problems with me. Nevertheless, my doctor still takes urinalysis, and still checks all those things."

"After I was diagnosed I read quite a bit about lupus," I said, "and I thought I was too old to get this disease. It strikes mostly young women in childbearing years."

"How old were you when you first had symptoms?"

"Well, it was in Hawaii; let's see, that would be . . . no, wait a minute, I had symptoms before I went to Hawaii, in my second marriage and even before then. That would make it in my thirties or earlier."

Dianne smiled and said, "In one of the recent lectures that we had, the doctor said that older people who still had the disease would probably have fewer and less severe episodes as their age advances. That was the best news I'd ever heard."

That was certainly the best news *I'd* heard in a long time! I thought.

"I read an article recently about people in the age 50-60 bracket who have lupus. Only one woman in 500 is diagnosed, because it's usually thought of as a disease hitting people in their childbearing years."

"Also, while it mainly hits women, men can be affected, as we know. And it's very hard on a man to suddenly become disabled this way."

"Amen!" Wally said. "Does anyone feel a bigger threat from the medications than from the disease? The end result of long-term medication?"

"Bigger threat or bigger fear?"

"I have a fear of what medications can do to me based on my past experiences," I said.

"I'm afraid of going off the medication," Mary said. "I fear not having anything for my body."

"I have strong feelings about the threat from medication," I said, remembering my Hawaii experience which I now briefly shared. "Still," I concluded, "it's saving a lot of people's lives. So even though I'm anti-medication for myself, I do know that it can do good when not misused by doctors and patients."

"I was on antimalarial, not for a life or death situation, but so that I could function. The medication enabled me to walk and function, so it wasn't a matter of life and death, but the quality of my life. But I was still frightened of the medication because I know what the side effects can do. Then, coming off the medication, I was afraid, too, afraid of not functioning. But I wanted so much to stop. The doctors warned me to do it slowly, so I wouldn't crash. So, I had the fear of coming off mixed with the fear of staying on."

". . . not knowing what to do!"

"Right, total fear and confusion. But now I'm elated. I didn't crash and for six months now, I have been in remission. That's the longest I've ever been off meds in four and a half years!"

"Well, I have to take about forty different pills daily, including calcium and vitamins and fourteen different prescriptions. I have a system where I put packets together for breakfast, lunch, dinner and bedtime. My ex-husband was putting together a week's worth of packets for me, but then I got so insecure, I had to start doing it myself."

"I thought you were in remission too."

"Yes, but I still have to take medications to keep me alive and in remission."

"Even in remission, the symptoms go on!"

"Fortunately, I'm not on any medication. Just last month there was a question of whether I'd have to go back on something. I'm trying it without, but it's been difficult. I've never found a medication my body and mind can tolerate and still function. Unfortunately, in my case, every medication is mind-altering for me. I get confused. I don't function as well,even though a lot of the pain and discomfort disappear. It just blows my mind, even the mildest anti-inflammatory."

"Each person is likely to have a different reaction to the same medication. The Clinoril that you're on, I can't function on. When they gave me that, I thought I would die. It's a non-steroid type of anti-inflammatory drug. I think I'd rather suffer the lupus than the effects that medication had on my body."

"Some of this stuff that we have to use is pretty potent. We're not talking about . . ."

"Yeah, I go to the pharmacy and he says in surprise, 'you're on that!' "

"And then there's plasmapheresis, when the blood is removed from a patient and replaced. I mean, this disease can subject you to all kinds of goodies!"

"Plasmapheresis was discussed with me. The doctor explained that it is the removal of plasma from withdrawn blood, with retransfusion of the formed elements into the donor. Usually, type-specific fresh frozen plasma or albumin is used to replace the withdrawn plasma. They also told me that if I develop another kidney problem, they'll use that instead of immunosuppressants."

"And then there's dialysis . . ."

"I had a call from a lady on dialysis who can't breathe without oxygen. Then the medication they used made her sick to her stomach and of course she couldn't take the oxygen to breathe when she was throwing up. So they're talking about plasmapheresis."

"It took a long time for me to tolerate the medication," Terry said. "I threw up and I was so sick."

"It's especially intolerable when you're throwing up

and trying to get oxygen to breathe!"

"I told the doctor that I was sick to my stomach, and he said that was part of kidney failure. That's fine! So I went through three months of daily vomiting—dry and wet heaves. Then, when I was hospitalized, I was all bloated, and when they tried to put a heparin lock in me, they couldn't find the vein. When I asked her how many times she'd punctured me, looking for it, there was no answer. Finally, I requested the head technician to draw the blood. You can't see anything when you're all bloated. So when she walked over to use my right arm, I said 'No way; get someone else.' Finally another technician came in, and she got it the first time."

"I'm careful about that stuff, too. If they don't find the vein the first time, I ask for someone else. I didn't used to think I could do that, but now I stand up for my rights. I've been punctured too many times. I also ask about checking meds when they give them to me. It's too easy to get the wrong drugs."

"That's happened with me too."

"It's important to know what drugs they're giving to you. Discuss it with your doctor. Then you have to ask the nurse what the drug is and what it's for before taking it. You can refuse a drug if there's a question."

"Once I started taking everything in the vein, I stopped vomiting. I started thinking, now what is going on! Hey, I'm going to put my prednisone in those jellied tubes! Then I was hospitalized in the mental section, and I started vomiting again from the pills. I wonder why, I asked myself—all of a sudden I'm taking all these pills and throwing up. I had to get out of there, and I became angry when they wanted to keep me longer. I felt strong enough to leave and as soon as I got home, I popped these in the jellied capsules and saved my own skin. I was going downhill and knew the med wasn't working because I was throwing it up. Now I could keep it down. So I don't know, we all have to be our own doctors, as well as finding a doctor we can work with. You're in a lot of trouble if you can't work with the doctor. Most doctors don't explain things so I can understand. They rattle off a lot of medical stuff. I don't know what they're talking about half the time."

"For some drugs, I've had to sign a release at the doctor's office that I was taking it."

"That's because the drug was experimental. Most of those drugs aren't anymore."

"It sure panics me when I have to sign a release form for drugs."

"What's a release form?"

"You sign that before the pharmacy gives you the prescription."

"You have to have faith in your doctor."

"Sure, but the doctor doesn't really know how a lot of things are going to affect me. So, I have to work with him and assume some of the responsibility."

"That's true."

"Everyone reacts differently. I was given Motrin and I started hallucinating."

"Me, too. Motrin made me crazy."

"I thought I was the only one!"

"All these drugs can cause reactions."

Two hours had gone by quickly. Once again, I was amazed at the honesty and knowledgeability of the people in the group, the openness and warm understanding. As I was preparing to leave, Claire asked me if I meditated.

"My favorite question to other people." I laughed. "But to answer you, yes I do. It helps with the pain and helps to relax me. You know, whatever works. I try most everything." That started others on the subject.

"I began doing self-hypnosis."

"I use a lot of self-hypnosis."

"I don't take any pain killers, so I have to do something," Terry said. "The other drugs help, but I'm still left with pain."

"The mind can be powerful in healing, too. I saw a show where two doctors spoke on this. While you may not cure anything with your mind, it can be an ally in the disease-fighting process, whether it be helping your immune system or whatever. Like with chemotherapy. Visualize the radiation doing its stuff, visualize the good thing it will accomplish, instead of the throwing up, and so on. Positive imagery."

"Right. That means that we can make whatever time we have better."

People were reluctant to leave, and I could hear other animated conversations—all going on at once.

"I have mitral valve prolapse," Wally said.

"I do too. Your doctor can usually hear some kind of clicking."

"I get terrible feelings of pressure, of suffocation."

"I had the suffocation," Terry said. "But it's clearing up. I would wake up suffocating. The air wasn't getting down there."

"And that's frightening in the middle of the night."

"There are so many weird things that happen. I can't even remember all of them. My memory is also going downhill. I used to be so happy-go-lucky. Now I have to just go with the flow on these things that happen."

"You accept it."

"It's like my mind is protecting me by not making a big deal about any of this, and then enabling me to forget how bad it was."

"The mind is a powerful thing," Dianne said. "And we can get it to work for us. Well gang, that's it for now. Thank you all for coming and sharing."

Before leaving the house, I turned to observe my friends. For long beautiful moments I stood there, drinking in the love and warmth that I sensed in the room. A smile started in my stomach and soared throughout my body. Then I turned around, slowly pressed the lever and the screen door squeaked open. I walked outside and a warm breeze filled me with excitement as I stepped out into the sunlight of a new day. For me, these rap sessions were highlights on the way to acceptance. I slept peacefully that night.

When I woke up the next morning I sensed a stillness in the room—and in me—that hadn't been there before. I had peace of mind. My head wasn't talking to me at a mile a minute. I felt free as never before. Then it came to me with sudden clarity—no matter what direction my health took, I was going to be all right. "Thank You, God," I prayed by the foot of my bed.

11

Acceptance

Now that I was home, one of the most difficult and tedious things to continue was the exercise plan from the hospital. In the beginning, I resented every second of the fifteen minutes that I spent twice a day doing the boring, tiring movements. But I kept at it anyway, taking care to neither overdo nor be lazy, as Pat had advised. Again, there was that trick of knowing how much was too much and how little was too little. But, whatever I did paid off in my feeling good. So on the days that I felt like quitting, I remembered to just slow down, not to stop altogether.

Before long, exercising became such a part of my daily routine that it was like brushing my teeth. On the days when fatigue and weakness took their toll on my body, I adjusted my exercise program to whatever I could handle. I'd begun to listen to my body, not my destructive thinking. How lucky I was to have been able to go to the arthritis rehabilitation program, I thought again, another addition to my grateful list. And I had brought along all those goodies, those special devices that made my life easier. I was thrilled to use them and wondered why *I* hadn't thought of things such as these!

I knew that I was conserving energy by following the hospital routines, and keeping my muscles and joints in good condition.

My two endurance exercises were walking and

swimming. I had begun walking while in the hospital, and now at home I was ready to expand on this, as well as to begin swimming every day again.

Just as with my diet regimen, my daughter Annie took an interest in my exercises. She sent me information about walking that served as a catalyst, prodding me into action with a walking program.

I bought a pair of walking shoes and thick absorbent socks and an earphone radio. I was ready to start this part of my wellness plan.

"It's not good to walk in heavy smog," Annie said. "You defeat your purpose when you breathe in all that junk. So try to walk in a park or someplace away from traffic."

I also kept in mind that I wasn't to rush my fitness program. I needed to work into it, not attempt to do it all in one day, as was my usual practice with something new. "Remember, pace yourself," I reminded myself. "Easy does it. Slow down!" That was still not easy for me, but at the rehabilitation hospital, the importance had somehow gotten my undivided attention. Something at the hospital had clicked for me and put it all together in my mind. It had worked there; it would work for me at home. So, one day at a time, I incorporated what I had learned into my daily living.

I planned my first walks to be short, but continuous. I would walk just for walking, not to get to the library or market or do other errands.

All set, with my earphone radio, I started out walking at a gentle pace for ten minutes every other day for the first week. At first I had to push myself to begin, but then, after a while, I looked forward to these walks. I loved being outdoors, and most of all I enjoyed the results. I felt more alive, less tense and irritable, and it was fun. I couldn't believe I felt that way. I wondered why I had waited so long to do it.

Annie had been strongly suggesting walking for years, and so had many of my friends, and also my son, who rarely imposed any suggestion on me. So, for the most part, I happily bounced to the street or park to walk, although there were still some days when I had to force myself into walking shoes and out the door. As I walked I became more interested in my surroundings. I nodded and smiled at other walkers, feeling myself a part of the widespread general interest in this type of exercise. Joggers sped by, but I knew that walking was better for me. It had most of the benefits of more strenuous exercise, and walking a mile burnt up just about as many calories as jogging at twice the walking speed. Was that information a surprise! I also learned that exercise will not increase hunger and result in weight gain, as I had feared. When the blood-sugar level drops, one feels hungry, but with exercise, the blood sugar remains stable because the muscles use more fat than sugar as fuel.

After the first week I gradually walked for longer periods, until in about six weeks I was walking forty minutes every other day. Each time I worked into my walking stints gradually and tapered off the same way in order to avoid soreness the next day.

"Don't forget to warm up before you start walking," Annie reminded me. "Also, when you stop walking, the muscles of the legs stop helping to return the blood to the heart, so remember to do your cooling down exercises at the end of a walk. And don't take a hot shower right after a walk, because the heat brings more blood to the skin and thus leaves less for the heart to pump to the vital organs."

Walking became the easiest and best exercise available for me, just as swimming was the best all-around body conditioner. So I walked. Even my body knew of my devotion to this form of exercise. At the end of just two weeks, I had become committed to a healthy and enjoyable pattern of exercising that even I could do.

"Rest is essential." I had heard this repeatedly, over and over at the hospital. It was just what my doctor had been telling me. Why had it been such trouble for me to incorporate periods of rest in my daily life? I knew the reason—I still felt guilty when I wasn't doing something productive. But I realized that I had to slow down or I wouldn't be able to produce anything at all, so I heeded those words and gave rest periods a chance.

Exercise and diet would not cure my chronic disease, but along with the many other healthy practices introduced to me at the hospital and now included in my life at home, they would increase my chances of living a longer, more productive, higher quality life. I had taken just one thing at a time, so I wouldn't feel overwhelmed by it all: eating correctly, walking, swimming and the countless other beneficial changes I was making. When I became accustomed to them, I found the routines took only an hour or so of each day. Surely I could spare that much time for something of such great importance.

I finally accepted the fact that I had lupus, but that did not mean that I was willing to give in to the disease. Along with my newfound serenity, I had also been given freedom of choice. I could decide the direction my life would take. I remembered reading about options that lupus patients had. It was in an excellent book titled, *Lupus Erythematosus, A Handbook For Nurses* by Terri Nass, R.N., and it said:

> The first choice is to submit to the disease and a lifestyle of illness as the new identity. This choice may appear attractive to a newly diagnosed patient who is exhausted from the long battle of uncertainties about her condition. However, this choice offers primarily a life of

> perpetual self-examination and may lead to self-pity or self-loathing. It will find its solace in further flares.
>
> The second choice is to fight the disease and create a different identity based upon reworked goals and expectations. Inherent within the second choice is greater control, greater self-image, and at the same time the potential for greater disappointment if goals and expectations have not been realistic, which may or may not be the fault of the patient.
>
> This latter choice requires imagination, resilience and spunk, and depends heavily upon an adequate support network which can buffer the disappointments that arise and encourage continued realistic goal-setting. This choice offers quality of life.

I chose the second way to live. Working realistically I pursued wellness, not illness. My goal could be expressed by the acronym HAPPY, meaning Health, Appearance, Peace of Mind, Perseverance and Youthful thinking. I kept HAPPY and HALT on my refrigerator door and imprinted on my mind, along with the words, Pace Yourself and Easy Does It.

I no longer was on a self-destructive path. I had hope for the future instead of despair, and peace of mind instead of confusion and fear. Even with lupus I was able to function one day at a time, and I enjoyed the prospect of continuing to live a quality life. Most of all, I loved the freedom I felt inside. What a joy that was!

Yes, I still have lupus. There is no cure. But today I do not allow the pain and manifestations of the disease to control my life. There was a time when I had chosen to die, and I was on the brink of death. But now, with God's help, I have won the battle in my mind. I have chosen to live, and I have chosen to be happy.

Related Support Organizations

American Chronic Pain Association
257 Old Haymaker Rd.
Monroeville, PA 15146
(412) 856-9676

American Lupus Society, The
23751 Madison Street
Torrance, CA 90505
(213) 373-1335
(800) 331-1802

Arthritis Foundation
1314 Spring Street, N.W.
Atlanta, GA 30309
(404) 872-7100

Lupus Foundation of America, Inc.
1717 Massachusetts Ave., N.W.
Suite 203
Washington, D.C. 20036
(202) 328-4550
(800) 558-0121

National Chronic Pain Outreach Association
4922 Hampden Lane
Bethesda, MD 20814
(301) 652-4948

Range of Motion Exercises

These are the exercises that I do which keep me mobile and enable me to maintain a positive attitude.

Beverly Brown

Courtesy of Daniel Freeman Memorial Hospital
In association with
Carondelet Rehabilitation Centers of America

Care must be taken to try to maintain what range of motion is present and possibly increase it. Daniel Freeman Memorial Hospital, in association with Carondelet Rehabilitation Centers of America has designed a program that goes through the range of motion of each joint of the body.

Range of motion is the distance a joint can move in a particular direction. Since arthritics tend to wake up stiff with decreased range of motion, and/or with pain in the morning, these exercises will obtain the best results if done in the morning. Doing it after a shower is even better, as the heat will help "loosen up" the muscles and ease up joint pain and stiffness.

Since arthritis does not take a day off, the range of motion exercises should be done daily, 365 days a year.

Do about 10 repetitions of each exercise. If you are in pain or have a flare-up, do the exercises, but decrease the repetitions to three or four.

Starting position: Sitting erect, looking straight ahead.

1. *Head Up/Head Down:* Tilt your head back as far as you can. Then try to bring your chin to your chest. Repeat.

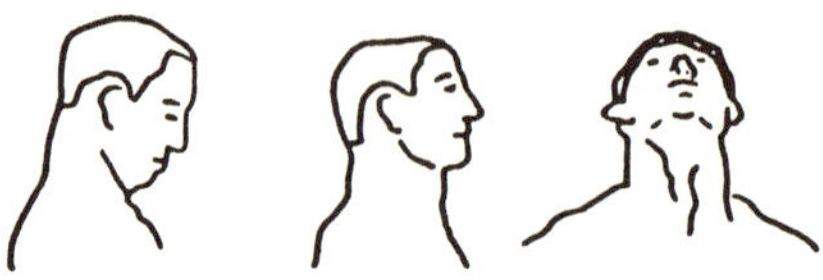

2. *Head Turns:* Turn your head to one side and look over your shoulder. Then turn it to the other side and look over that shoulder. Repeat.

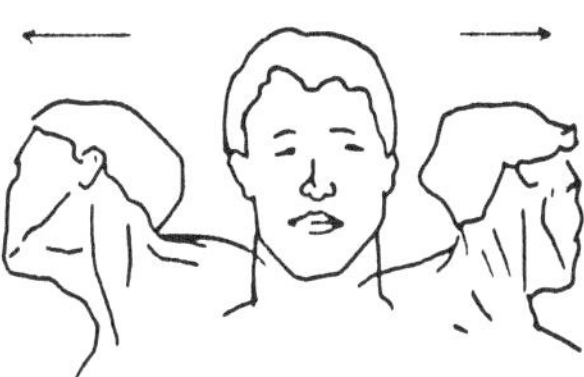

3. *Ear to Shoulder:* Bring your ear to your shoulder. Then bring your other ear to your other shoulder. Do not lift the shoulder when moving your head. Repeat.

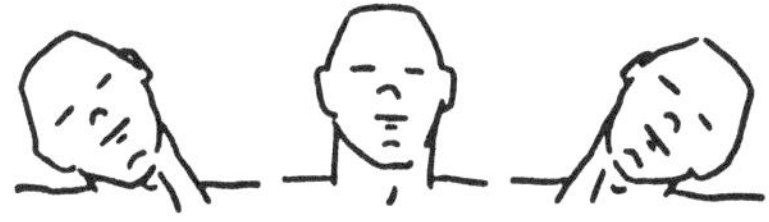

4. *Shoulder Shrugs:* Shrug your shoulders to your ears as high as you can. Then let your shoulders down. Repeat.

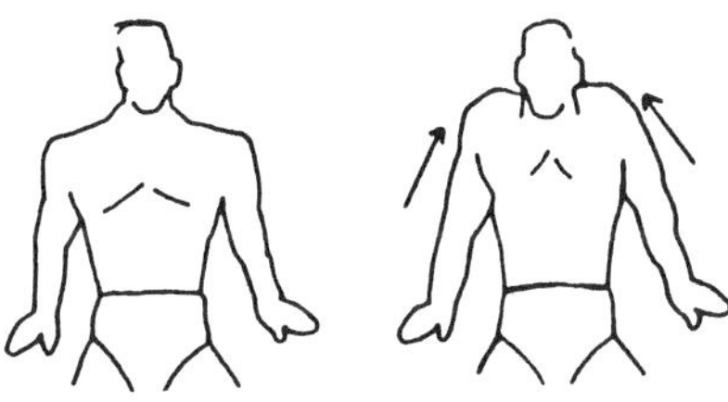

5. *Arm Circles:* Raise your arms out to the side at shoulder level. Make a circle forward with your arms. Repeat. Then make circles in the opposite direction in the same way.

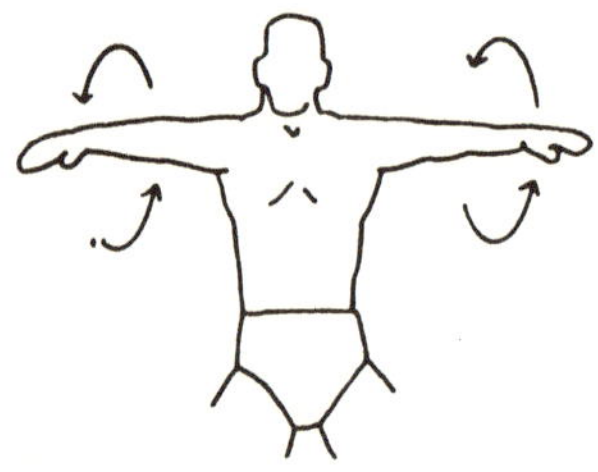

6. *Butterfly:* Grasp your hands behind your neck with your elbows pointing out towards the sides. Bring your elbows together, and then move them out to the sides again. Repeat.

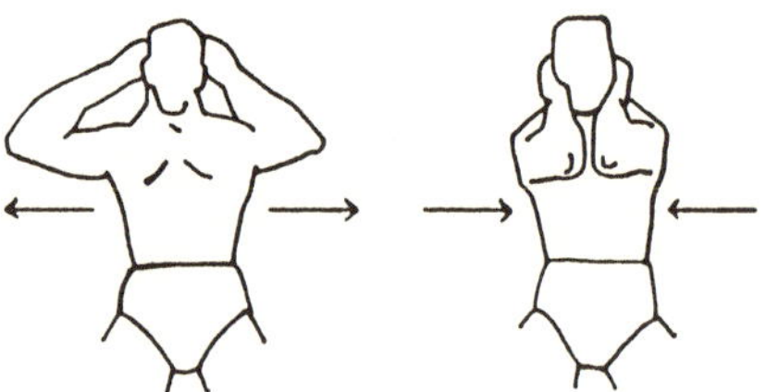

Alternate Butterfly: Bend your elbows with your hands pointing up at the ceiling. Bring your elbows and hands together, and then move them back out to the sides again. Repeat.

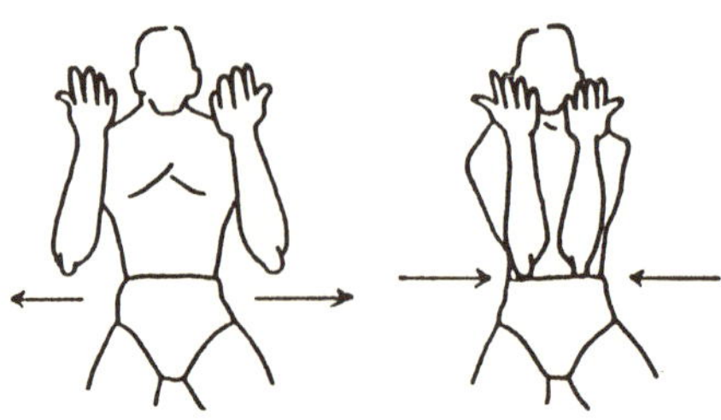

7. *Reach Behind Back:* Start with your arms straight out in front of you, with your palms facing out. Reach behind your back. Then reach up towards your shoulder blades and back down. Bring your hands back together in front. Repeat.

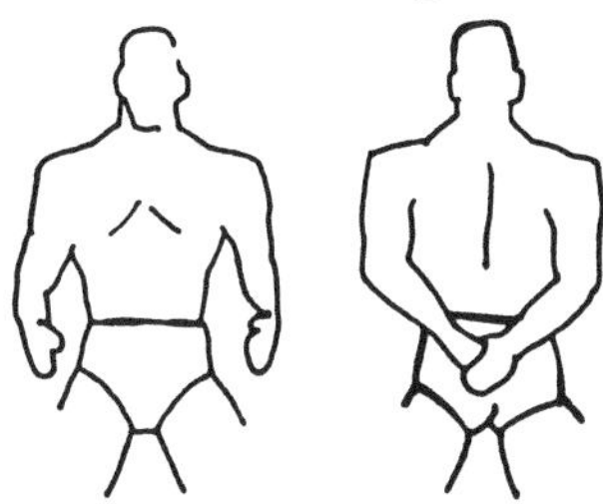

8. *Elbow Bends:* Bend your elbows by touching your fingertips to your shoulders. Then straighten out your arms completely. Repeat.

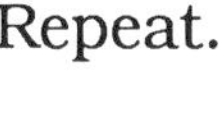

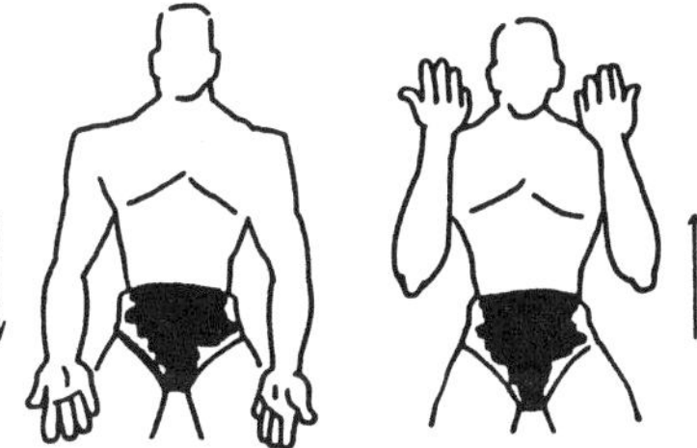

9. *Palms Up/Palms Down:* Start with your elbows bent at your side and your palms facing down. Next, flip your palms up. Flip them back down again. Repeat.

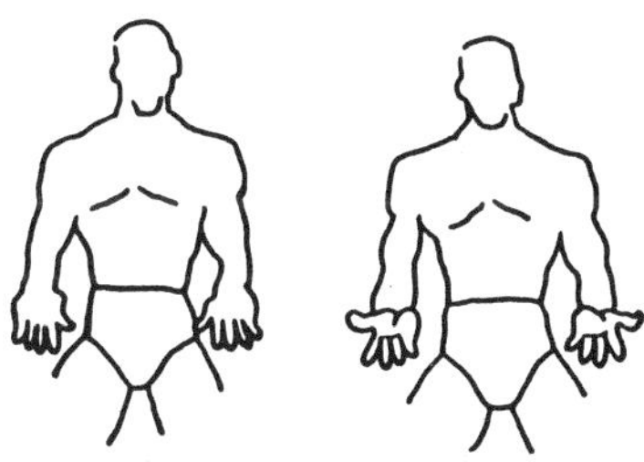

10. *Wrist Bends:* With your elbows bent at your side and your palms facing down, bend your wrists up and then down. Only your wrists should be moving. Repeat.

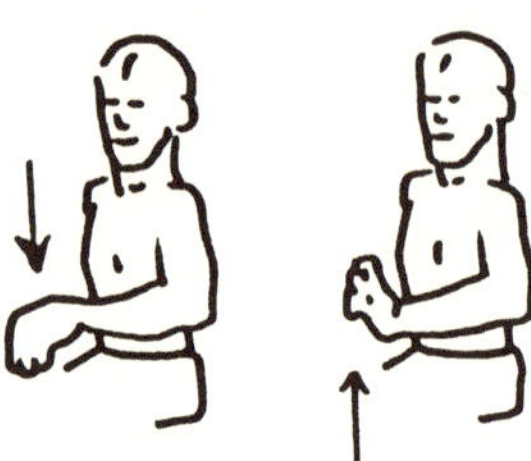

11. *Open and Close Hands:* Make a fist with both hands. Then open up your hands with all your fingers completely straight. Repeat.

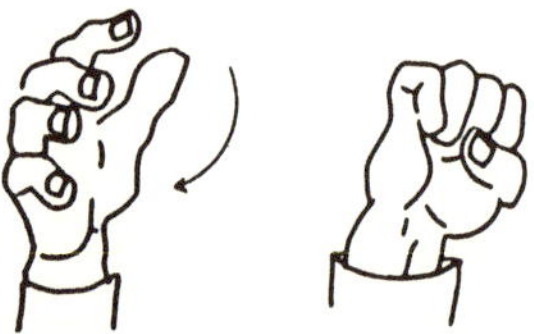

12. *Finger to Thumb:* Make an "O" by touching your thumb to your finger tip. Touch each finger in the same way one by one.

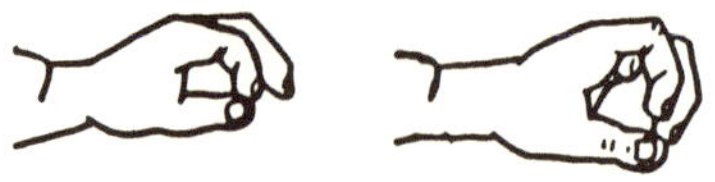

13. *Ankle Circles:* Move your feet in a circle. Repeat. Then move your feet in a circle in the opposite direction in the same way.

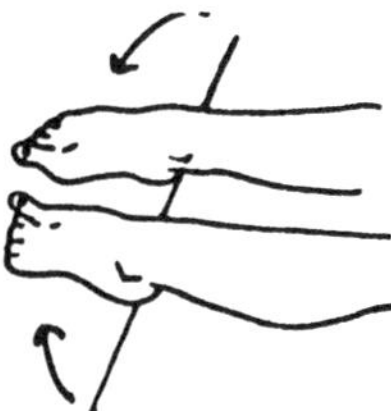

14. *Sidebends:* Lean to one side and then to the other side. Repeat. Starting position: Seated or standing.

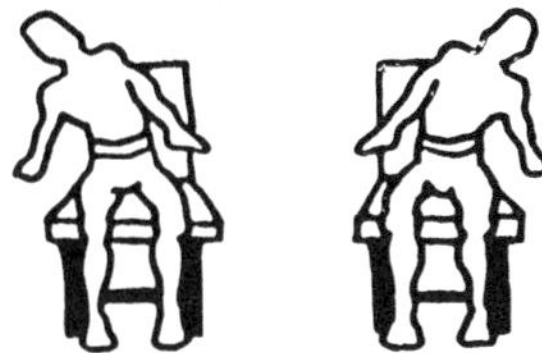

15. *Straight Leg Raises:* Lie with one knee bent and the foot flat on the mat, and the other leg straight. Keeping your knee straight, lift it up towards the ceiling to the level of your other knee. Lower it down slowly. Repeat. Do the same thing with the other leg.

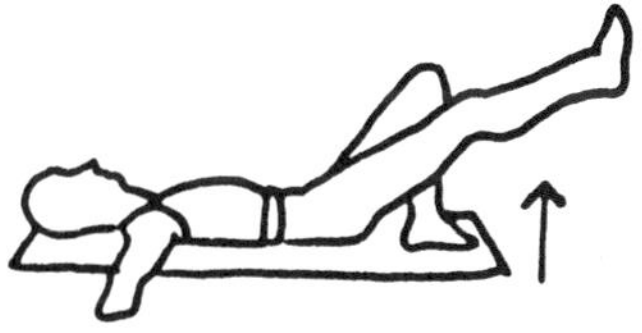

16. *Knee to Chest:* Lie with both knees bent and both feet flat on the mat. Bring one knee up to your chest as far as possible. Then lower it back down slowly. Next, bring the other knee up in the same way. Repeat.

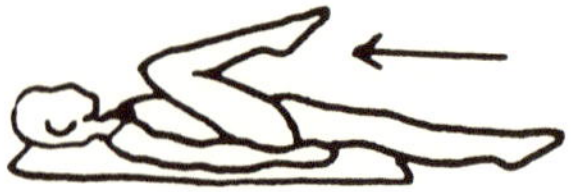

17. *Bridges:* Lie with both knees bent and both feet flat on the mat. Lift your buttocks up high in the air and then lower it down slowly. Repeat.

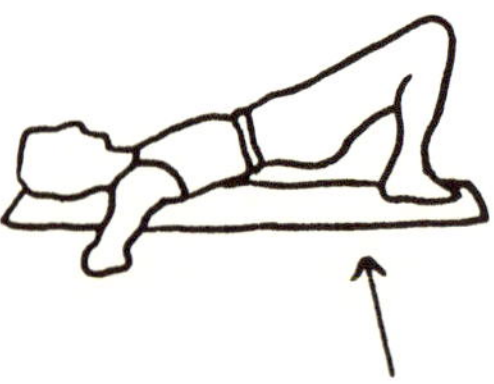

18. *Partial Sit Ups:* Both knees bent and both feet flat on the mat. Cross your arms over your chest. Now lift your head and shoulders up off the mat. Then lower yourself back down slowly. Repeat.

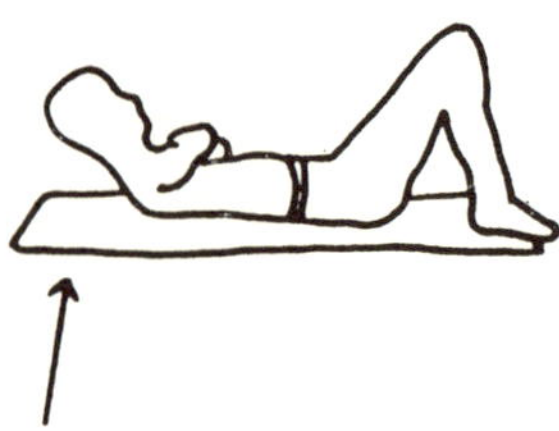

19. *Arm Raises:* Lie with both arms at your side. Slowly lift one arm over your head as far back as it will go. Then lower it back down to your side. Next, lift the other arm over your head in the same way. Repeat.

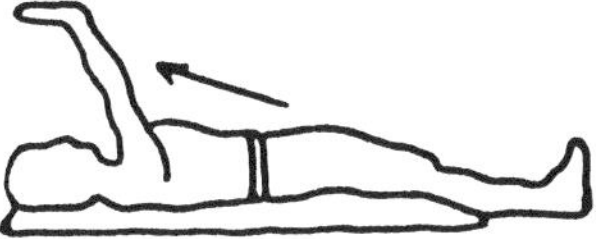

20. *Side Leg Lifts:* Lie on your side with the bottom leg bent for balance and the top leg straight. Keeping the leg straight, lift it up towards the ceiling as high as you can. Then lower it down slowly. Repeat. Be sure you are not rolled forward, but on your side. Now turn over and lift the other leg.

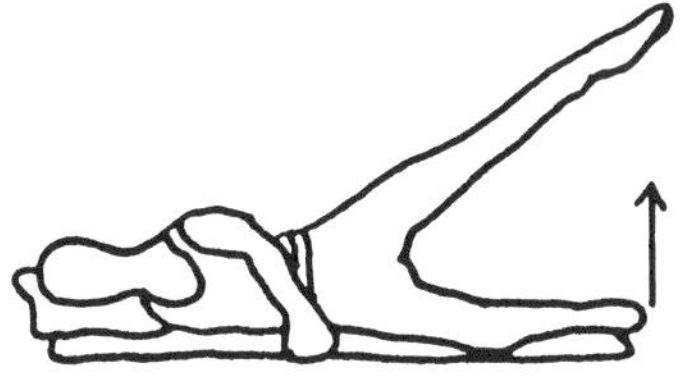

Alternate Side Leg Lifts: Lie on your back. Keeping your leg straight, bring leg out to the side. Then bring it back in. Repeat.

21. *Back Leg Lifts:* Lie on your stomach. You can put a small towel roll at your forehead so your neck is straight. Keeping your knee straight, lift your leg straight up towards the ceiling as high as you can get it. Lower it back down slowly. Repeat. Then lift your other leg in the same way.

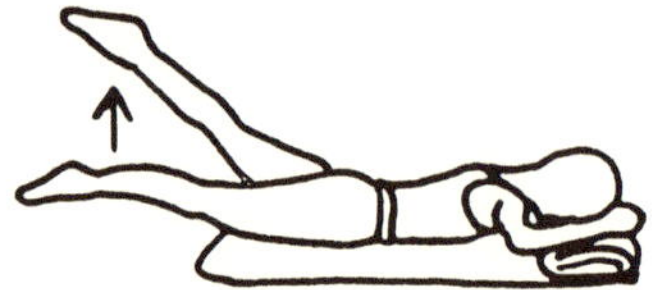

22. *Quad Sets:* Lie on your back with both legs straight. Tighten the knees (quad muscles) by pushing the back of your knees down into the mat. Hold it for five counts. Repeat.

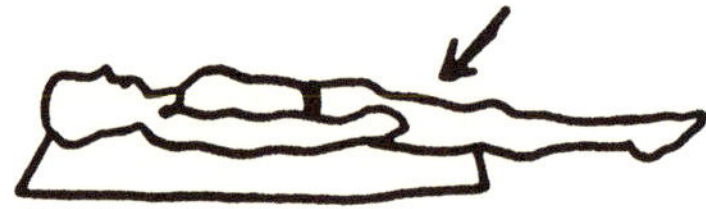

23. *Glut Sets:* Lie on your back with both legs straight. Tighten your buttock muscles (glut muscles) by squeezing them together. Hold it for five counts. Repeat.

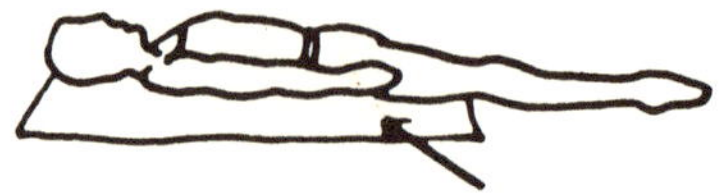